FROM COMMUNITY CARE
TO MARKET CAR

Dedication
Lyn Harrison 1941–2001
We wish to dedicate this book to a close colleague, good friend and indomitable spirit.

FROM COMMUNITY CARE TO MARKET CARE?

The development of welfare services for older people

Robin Means, Hazel Morbey and Randall Smith

The POLICY

PRESS

First published in Great Britain in April 2002 by

The Policy Press
34 Tyndall's Park Road
Bristol BS8 1PY
UK

Tel +44 (0)117 954 6800
Fax +44 (0)117 973 7308
e-mail tpp@bristol.ac.uk
www.policypress.org.uk

British Library Cataloguing in Publication Data

A catalogue record for this book is available from the British Library

ISBN 1 86134 265 9 paperback

A hardcover version of this book is also available

Robin Means is Associate Dean (Research and International Developments) and
Hazel Morbey is a Research Associate, both at the Faculty of Health and Social Care
at the University of the West of England in Bristol. **Randall Smith** is a Senior
Research Fellow at the School for Policy Studies, University of Bristol.

Cover design by Qube Design Associates, Bristol.

Photograph on front cover supplied by www.johnbirdsall.co.uk

Printed and bound in Great Britain by Hobbs the Printers Ltd, Southampton.

Contents

List of tables and figures

Tables

Figures

Advisory Group members

Paul Bywaters   Head of Social Work, Coventry University

David Gladstone   Senior Lecturer in Social Policy, University of Bristol

Gordon Lishman   Operations Director (now Director General), Age Concern, England

Rodney Lowe   Professor of Historical Studies, University of Bristol

Ian White, CBE   Director of Social Services, Hertfordshire County Council, 1995-2000

Acknowledgements

This study was made possible by a generous grant from the Economic and Social Research Council (Grant No R000 23 7279). In addition, we are indebted to the staff, past and present, of the four local authorities that inspired our case studies. Thanks are especially due to those key players who agreed to be interviewed. We were well supported by our Advisory Group members. The presentation of our argument was enhanced by the experienced staff of The Policy Press and by suggestions for improving the text by two anonymous readers. We would also like to acknowledge the secretarial support received from Bernadette Cox, Deb Joy, Sandy Green and Leigh Taylor from the Faculty of Health and Social Care, University of the West of England (Bristol). Inadequacies are, of course, our responsibility.

Robin Means
Hazel Morbey
Randall Smith

ONE

Setting the scene

Background to the book

The UK government's approach to meeting the health and welfare needs of older people continues to be highly contentious, despite the publication of a national service framework for older people (DoH, 2001b). For example, one response has been a report calling for 'a new social compact for care in old age' (Robinson, 2001). It would mean that we are as uncertain as ever about the health and social care divide, the appropriate role of long-term care and how best to fund services. This book contributes to these contemporary debates by reflecting critically on the long historical roots of these issues and the difficulties faced in throwing off the legacy of the past.

This book is in many ways a sequel to *From Poor Law to community care: The development of welfare services for elderly people, 1939-71* (Means and Smith, 1985, 1998a). This was originally published by Croom Helm in the mid-1980s, but a much later second edition was produced by The Policy Press. The earlier book traced the roots of all those services, which were to become the responsibility of social services authorities from 1 April 1971, and had at its core an exploration of the long history of neglect of services for older people. The new book continues the story through to the implementation on 1 April 1993 of the main community care changes introduced by the 1990 National Health Service and Community Care Act.

The assumption of both books is that the study of contemporary history can illuminate the present, and that it can do this by helping us to sharpen our appreciation of the continuities and discontinuities of present policy and practice with the past. The early 21st century is a very good time to reassess the necessity for such long-term perspectives, which are not underpinned by myths of either the golden age of municipal socialism or the evils of Thatcherite privatisation. The Labour government elected in May 1997 initially appeared to have a modest programme of welfare reforms (Means and Smith, 1998b), but this has proved to be far from the case because of a modernisation agenda every bit as complex and far-reaching as the privatisation and quasi-market reforms of Conservative governments during the 1980s and 1990s. This modernisation agenda encompasses social protection policies (DSS, 1998), local government (Deputy Prime Minister, 1998), social services (DoH, 1998a), the National Health Service (DoH, 1997), as well as central government (Prime Minister, 1999).

This modernisation agenda is having a major impact on the availability of health and social care services for older people. It is also clear that community care for older people remains a critical policy issue, as can be seen in the government response (Secretary of State for Health, 2000b) to the far-reaching recommendations of the Royal Commission on Long-Term Care (Sutherland Report, 1999). This debate reflects the public expenditure implications of an ageing society and continuing concerns about the role of the state in meeting the health and social care needs of frail elders.

The Griffiths Report and the reform of community care

Chapter Two focuses on the modernisation agenda of the Labour government and the relevance of a grasp of contemporary history to an understanding of present day challenges. However, the genesis of the book was not the community care debates of the early years of the new millennium, but rather the debates of the mid-1990s about the strengths and weaknesses of the community care reforms called for by the Griffiths Report (1988), outlined in the subsequent White Paper (DoH, 1989a) and broadly implemented through the 1990 NHS and Community Care Act.

The restructuring of welfare provision in the 1980s and early 1990s was based on a critique of the inefficiency and ineffectiveness of previous provision with its heavy reliance upon the state as both purchaser and provider of services (Gladstone, 1995; Le Grand and Bartlett, 1993). With regard to community care, a series of reports (for example, the Firth Report, 1987; House of Commons Social Services Committee, 1985; National Audit Office, 1987) provided ammunition for those calling for a radical overhaul of provision. Key difficulties exposed included the lack of responsiveness on the part of local authority services, failures of joint working between health and social services and the mushrooming cost of paying for people to live in independent sector residential and nursing homes through the social security budget.

The most influential commentary was provided by the Audit

Commission (1986) report, *Making a reality of community care*, which criticised the very slow movement of people with mental health problems, people with learning difficulties and older people from hospital to community-based provision. The report concluded that progress towards community care for these groups had been far too slow, geographically uneven and that far too many people had been moved into independent sector residential or nursing home care, rather than into community-based provision. The report identified five underlying problems:

- *Mismatch of resources:* funds for community care came from numerous sources and were uncoordinated.
- *The lack of a bridging fund:* a transition fund was needed so that community services could be built up before hospitals were closed.
- *Perverse effects of social security policy:* health and local authorities could access social security funds to meet care costs if the person was in residential or nursing home care, but not if they were living in the community (and access to benefit was not based upon an assessment of need).
- *Organisational fragmentation and confusion:* many agencies were involved in community care and it was not clear which was the lead agency between health and social services.
- *Inadequate staffing.*

The main response of the government to the critique by the Audit Commission was to establish a review of community care chaired by Sir Roy Griffiths. As outlined in earlier work (Means and Smith, 1998b), four main themes dominated the report:

- that for thirty years central government had failed to develop any link between the objectives of community care policy and the resources made available to meet those objectives;
- that responsibilities at the local level were unclear between health authorities, social services authorities, housing authorities, the voluntary sector and the private sector, and coordination was not well developed;
- that choice and efficiency should be stimulated through a mixed economy approach in which the public, private and voluntary sectors competed to provide services on an equal footing;
- that the system of subsidising private and voluntary sector residential and nursing home places through the social security system was wasteful because of the lack of assessment of need for residential care.

A key recommendation in the Griffiths Report (1988) was that social services authorities should be the lead agency for all the main community care groups including older people because such authorities are grounded in the community and accountable to democratically elected councillors. However, social services were not being asked to dominate service provision, but rather to continue to develop a mixed economy of provision. This was to be guided by care management and assessment at the micro/individual level and by a new system of annual community care plans at the macro/strategic level.

Funding and assessment for independent sector residential and nursing home care were to be transformed. Through assessment by care managers, social services would explore with the client whether or not community based or institutional care was the best option. For those who entered a residential or nursing home after this process, social services would meet their care costs subject to a means test. A transfer of social security monies to social services would enable this to happen and those monies would effectively have an annual limit for each local authority so that the public expenditure bill for such care would cease to rise in the dramatic fashion of the past.

The Conservative government made no formal response to the Griffiths Report, but many felt it was dismayed by its emphasis on the pivotal role of local authorities (Baldwin and Parker, 1989; Means and Smith, 1998b). However, it was difficult for the government to generate alternative organisational arrangements such as some kind of joint health/social services board and there was an urgent need to control social security expenditure on private residential and nursing home care (Hudson, 1990; Lewis and Glennerster, 1996). As a result, the White Paper on *Caring for people: Community care in the next decade and beyond* (DoH, 1989a) broadly followed the recommendations of Sir Roy Griffiths and endorsed his vision of social services authorities "as arrangers and purchasers of care services rather than as monopolistic providers" (p 17). This was seen as involving three main roles:

- carrying out an appropriate assessment of an individual's need for social care (including residential and nursing home care) and in collaboration as necessary with medical, nursing and other caring agencies, before deciding what services should be provided;
- designing packages of services tailored to meet the assessed needs of individuals and their carers. The appointment of a 'case manager' could facilitate this;

• securing the delivery of services, not simply by acting as direct providers, but by developing a purchasing and contracting role to become "enabling authorities" (p 17).

In addition, the White Paper confirmed a new funding structure for independent sector residential and nursing homes, with local authorities becoming responsible for financing the care support of people in such homes over and above their entitlement to general social security benefits.

Reactions to the White Paper were less favourable on the whole than to the Griffiths Report. Hudson (1990) attacked the White Paper and the subsequent 1990 Act as an expedient way to cap social security payments. Both Langan (1990) and Biggs (1990/91) perceived them very much in terms of the 'marketisation' of welfare. Walker (1989) saw them as the starting point for a greater reliance on charging and self-provisioning than had been the case before.

More recent commentators expressed greater hostility, a point that we reflected on in Chapter One of the revised edition of our previous study:

> ... the message of many commentators is one of *Care in Chaos* (Hadley and Clough, 1996) as local authorities struggle to meet their expanded responsibilities within available resources. A key feature of these critiques is often a comparison of the limitations of the market ideology of the 1990 reforms (efficiency and consumer responsiveness coming from providers competing for 'business') with the more welfare-orientated ideology of the past with its emphasis on a right to free services. Thus, Dominelli and Hoogvelt (1996) complain of the move in social work from needs-led to budget-led provision and from the direct provision of services to the managing of services provided by others. (Means and Smith, 1998a, p 1)

However, such perspectives were in marked contrast to those, mainly from the right, who felt that consumer orientated community care could never be generated unless the role of local authorities was severely curtailed and privatisation pushed much further than allowed under the 1990 Act.

The Economic and Social Research Council (ESRC) study on which this book is based was designed to challenge both the proponents and the critics of the community care reforms. The reforms had been partly justified by reference to the deficiencies of local authority run services in the 1970s and 1980s, yet surprisingly little research had concentrated upon policy and practice debates at the local level, including the interplay of factors that might have restricted the ability of local authorities to develop a flexible range of community care services for older people. Equally, critics of the reforms seemed sometimes to drift into what Pearson (1983) called the 'myth of the golden age', which in community care terms meant a time when free services were supposed to be available to all older people as a right. This was manifestly not the case with charging, rationing and service provision by the voluntary sector all very much part of the community care landscape from the late 1940s onwards (Means and Smith, 1998a).

The rationale for the study, therefore, lay in the contribution that analysing the development of community care services could make to understanding the strengths and weaknesses of the reform of community care that took place in the early 1990s. Chapter Two shows that it is equally valid to apply the same logic to illuminate policy issues and dilemmas generated by the modernisation policies of subsequent Labour governments. Before this can be done, however, it is necessary to describe the research study in more detail, together with some of the methodological challenges it posed.

Research objectives and methodology

The research team's aim was to chart how the development of welfare services for older people in England between 1971 and 1993 reflected changing assumptions about the roles of the public, private, voluntary and informal sectors in the provision of social support for older people. In particular, how did these assumptions influence policy and practice developments at the local level? The main objectives of the research were as follows:

• to outline the development of welfare services for older people from 1971 to 1993;
• to explore whether service developments in this period were as inadequate as claimed by the proponents of radical change;
• to identify both the continuities and the changes in the pre and post 1990 Act systems of community care;
• to draw upon the community care debates from 1971 to 1993 to illustrate contemporary concerns about such key issues as paying for care and the health and social care divide.

Unlike the earlier 1939-71 study, the research strategy for this project was based on a case study approach using four contrasting local authorities – a London Borough (Case Study A), two English Counties (Case Studies

B and C) and a Metropolitan Authority (Case Study D) – that had featured in earlier work undertaken by Means and his colleagues (Hoyes et al, 1993, 1994). Documentary material from key local agencies was of central importance, supplemented by interviews with key players. The kinds of documents scrutinised tended to be those officially in the public arena, such as reports to meetings of the Social Services Committees of the case study areas. The research team began by scrutinising Social Services Committee reports for the 22 year period in the four case study areas. (There were minor difficulties in accessing the records for the years 1971 to 1974 for those authorities affected by local government reorganisation in the early 1970s.)

The Social Services Committee reports proved to be a useful source for identifying other relevant documents, such as reports, annual or otherwise, of relevant local voluntary bodies, such as Age Concern or the Women's Royal Voluntary Service. However, documentary material was patchy from these kinds of sources. NHS records proved to be difficult to trace and a decision was taken, on the grounds of time and the large amount of material that was easily accessible, to rely on those relevant NHS reports on services for older people that were available in local authority or voluntary sector archives or that were provided by key informants. Other useful documents included commissioned local studies on services for older people. The documentation (and, indeed, the views of key players) was not seen as unproblematic. The research team tried to recognise the purposes of the reports scrutinised and to understand why some issues were initially raised but not pursued in the documentation. Apparent contradictions between different sources were seen as potentially illuminating rather than merely puzzling (Scott, 1990; Silverman, 1995).

In designing the study, the research team tried to follow the collective case study approach (Stake, 1995). The selection of the four case study areas was based on 'balance, variety and the opportunity to learn'. The four localities were varied and contrasting in terms of geography, type of local authority and management styles. The opportunity to learn was, as already hinted, based in part on previous successful work in these areas and the willingness of key gatekeepers to allow the team to do further work in the area.

This system of selecting the case studies hit one, unexpected snag. One of the four areas had destroyed its committee records such that they were available only from the mid-1980s.

The difficulty in tracing NHS records and the destruction of committee records in one of the four case study areas originally selected should be a matter of great concern to the former Department of the Environment,

Transport and the Regions, which was responsible for the main legislation relating to records in local authority custody, and more broadly to the Museums, Libraries and Archives Council, the National Council on Archives, the Association of Chief Archivists in Local Government and, in central government, the Inter-Departmental Archives Committee. The publication late in 1999 of government policy on archives should help to ensure that local authorities and other bodies providing a public service do invest appropriately in the preservation of invaluable records (Lord Chancellor, 1999).

In relation to the case study area with inadequate records, after some reflection and negotiation, another local authority of the same type and in the same area was identified to become Case Study D and agreed to participate. However, its history of management style was different from that of the local authority it replaced. By way of compensation, it had developed a corporate strategy in respect to older people as early as the mid-1970s, and this corporate strategy extended to include the voluntary sector. In that sense it provided a rich source of data for the early as well as the later years of the period of study.

Even though only four localities were to be studied, the research team was aware that there was likely to be an enormous mass of material to collect, process and analyse. How were decisions to be taken on what to include and what to exclude? The team decided that the overall study should have a thematic focus, and should not be made up of individual local studies. Based on their previous work (Means and Smith, 1985, 1998a) and their awareness of the work of others, a list of themes was devised and subsequently refined in consultation with the members of the Advisory Group. Some of the themes were listed in the fourth objective of the research (paying for care, the health and social care divide). Others included (i) institutional care for older people; (ii) the mixed economy of social care; (iii) who should get what? (rationing and prioritisation); and (iv) interagency and interprofessional working.

The identification of key players in each locality was initially informed by past work in three of the four case study areas and partly by the research team's familiarity with the policy field. The detailed scrutiny of documentation provided further leads. For the years 1971-72, 1981-82 and 1991-92 an attempt was made to identify the relevant Directors and Deputy Directors of Social Services and Chairs of Social Services Committees, and senior staff closely involved in services for older people, key players from the NHS side, (using the main Joint Consultative Committee documents appended to Social Services Committee reports) and from local voluntary and other bodies, such as Age Concern or the

Community Health Council, leading representatives from local trades unions and professional association branches and people from organisations of older people themselves. The attempt to identify key trades union and professional association people was less than successful. In all, 39 people were interviewed and their views were tape recorded.

Introducing the rest of the book

As outlined in the previous section, the book is organised around key themes relating to the future of community care for older people. Chapter Two, therefore, explores the community care and modernisation agenda of the 1997-2001 Labour government. Chapter Three explores the history of targeting and rationing domiciliary services for older people, while Chapter Four examines the long running issue of residential care for older people. The focus of Chapter Five is another long-standing theme – the shifting boundaries between what is deemed to be social care as opposed to health care. Chapter Six addresses moves to establish a mixed economy of social care, while Chapter Seven focuses on the community care reforms in terms of the attempt to establish what Le Grand and others have called quasi-markets (Le Grand and Bartlett, 1993). Chapter Eight offers reflections on continuity and change in the light of the modernisation agenda of the re-elected Labour government and possible lessons for the development of effective and user-centred community care policies in the early years of the new century.

The approach is, therefore, thematic in which illustrative examples are drawn from the case studies rather than the case studies being presented in detail in their own right. Nor is there an attempt to draw out the complexities of local political change and how this impacted in detail on the direction of community policy and practice within each of the four local authorities. The length of period under study would have made this an unrealistic objective within the resources available to the research team. Instead this book aims to give a strong flavour of the broad debates that occurred and some of the key influences and assumptions that lay behind those debates. The heavy reliance on reports to Social Services Committees and on interviews with senior social services managers means that there is almost certainly a managerial bias to the views presented. However, we still feel this provides a crucial counterbalance to the superficiality about the past that exists in most contemporary debates about community care.

Establishing social services in the early 1970s

Unified social services departments came into being on 1 April 1971 as a result of the recommendations of the Seebohm Report (1968) and the subsequent 1970 Local Authority Social Services Act. The new departments combined the previous work of children's departments and welfare departments, as well as much of the mental health functions of local authority health departments. Social services departments were to be headed by Directors of Social Services and their areas of responsibility with regard to older people included local authority residential homes, the home help service, meals and lunch club provision, laundry facilities, aids and adaptations and social work/counselling services.

It can be seen from the above that the book does not devote a chapter to the early social services departments in the first half of the 1970s in the same way that Chapter Seven addresses the detailed planning required by the community care changes of the early 1990s. One reason for this was the very fragmented nature of the available material, as much of the key planning occurred in the years immediately prior to the beginning of the study period. What does come across is the extent to which resources were stretched, especially in terms of the availability of qualified social workers and experienced managers, combined with the enormous challenge of blending the different components that needed to be brought together in the new departments (see also Means and Smith, 1998a, Chapter Seven). This often called for difficult priority decisions. For example, the London Borough was quite clear that priority had to be given to the establishment of a coherent childcare service[1] before the development of community care provision.

In respect of these early years, however, it is important to stress how the Metropolitan Authority stood out as strikingly different. It established a working group that included representation from the health service (interview with health visitor [D], 1971-87) and the voluntary sector (interview with General Secretary, Council of Voluntary Service [D], 1973-81), with a remit:

> ... to examine the total needs of, and provision for, the elderly in the Metropolitan Borough, and to advise the Council on all future provision in this field[2].

The working group covered housing/accommodation, domestic services, social contact and leisure activities, health and poverty[3]. As such, the authority was taking a corporate approach to planning that recognised the need for a partnership with other agencies and the wide determinants of the health and well being of older people. A corporate planner from that period stressed that the early 1980s had seen a number of local authorities, including this case study, attempting a corporate rational planning approach designed to challenge narrow departmental boundaries and based on the assessment of need at an area level (interview with corporate planner [D], 1973-76).

The working group was established in a period of optimism about public expenditure growth and so, as the corporate planner remembered, it was "uplifting to us group of officers", since "people [came] to the table, feeling buoyed up that they were going to be going away from the table with expansions in their services" (interview with corporate planner [D], 1973-76). However, the final report of the group was not available until 1976[4] by which time a period of financial stringency had arrived (see Chapters Three and Four). This forced the group to argue that additional investment in domiciliary services would need to be at the cost of "lower priority for expenditure on current forms of residential and geriatric in patient care", and that the priority for resources in the next three years needed to be "the group of the elderly with the most intense problems who are living in the community"[5]. Chapters Three and Four will illustrate how the Metropolitan Authority found it difficult to tackle this challenging agenda and how the other three case studies faced similar dilemmas.

Nevertheless, the fact that this authority had a broader vision about the breadth of their responsibilities for older people needs to be noted, as well as their commitment to improve services through partnerships with the health and the voluntary sector, especially since strong elements of this are to be found in the modernisation agenda of recent Labour governments (see Chapters Two and Eight). Indeed, the authority stands out because of the innovative nature of this vision. The rest of the book will show how all four case studies tried hard to improve community care services for older people, but that this was rarely attempted with any sense of a clear and creative vision, either from within the local authority or from central government.

Notes

[1] Social Services Committee (A), 13 September 1971 (Interim Report on Strategy Needs in Homes for the Elderly).

[2] Policy and Resources Committee (D), 30 October 1974 (The Elderly: An Interim Report).

[3] Ibid.

[4] Metropolitan Authority (D), March 1976 (The Elderly: A Policy Report).

[5] Ibid.

TWO

Community care and the modernisation of welfare

Introduction

There have been massive shifts in the public policy agenda since the research that underpins this book was first mooted in the mid-1990s. The Conservative Party lost the 1997 election and hence their pursuit of ever more privatised and market oriented forms of welfare provision were called into question. Although the Labour Party fought the election with the slogan of the 'Third Way', it was not immediately apparent what the implications of this were to be for the welfare state in general (Powell, 1999) or community care in particular (Means and Smith, 1998b).

Manifesto commitments relating to community care were limited, but included the following:

- civil rights to be developed for disabled people;
- a long-term care charter to define standards;
- independent inspection and regulation for residential and domiciliary care;
- a Royal Commission to establish a fair system for funding long-term care.

Although implying something of a rights-based approach to community care for older people, Means and Smith (1998b, p 239) pointed out that "such optimism has to be tempered by the fact that the two biggest manifesto commitments of all were not to raise the basic rate of income tax and not to exceed the public expenditure plans of the previous administration for the next two years".

Although these financial restrictions proved to be as limiting as feared, it did not stop a wide range of policy documents being published, which set out a radical reform agenda for the welfare state. In addition, the end of the two year public expenditure limit saw the Labour government in a position to invest considerable extra public expenditure on health and welfare services. In its July 1998 Local Authority Social Services Letter (98)13, the Department of Health announced the outcome of the Comprehensive Spending Review. Additional resources for the National Health Service (NHS) in England over the three year period 1999-2000 to 2001-02 amounted to £17.7 billion, and for the personal social services there was to be an additional £2.8 billion.

This chapter sets out the main components of this modernisation agenda as the key context for the empirical chapters of the book. The final chapter will draw the two strands together by reflecting on whether or not the new policy framework is as radical and different as claimed by the government.

Meeting manifesto commitments

It could be argued that the government managed to meet all its manifesto commitments. In terms of disability, a Disability Rights Commission was established, backed up by the additional rights established through the 1995 Disability Discrimination Act. From April 2002, a new system of standards for long-term care was brought in as a result of the 2000 Care Standards Act, which covers issues such as accommodation choice, access to health and social care, staffing levels, complaints systems and the availability of social activities. These standards are to be implemented and monitored through the National Care Standards Commission. The Commission is to take over local authority inspection and regulation units and be responsible for residential and nursing homes, children's homes, domiciliary care agencies, adoption and fostering agencies, as well as private and voluntary hospitals.

However, the highest profile manifesto commitment was without doubt the establishment of a Royal Commission on the funding of long-term care. Sir Stewart Sutherland was asked to chair the Commission. Its remit was:

> ... to examine the short and long term options for a sustainable system of funding of Long Term Care for elderly people, both in their own homes and in other settings, and within 12 months, to recommend how and in what circumstances the cost of such care should be apportioned between public funds and individuals. (Sutherland Report, 1999, p ix)

The decision to establish such a Commission reflected growing criticism of how the capital resources (and especially the home equity) of older people was being consumed in the last few years of life through expenditure on nursing and residential care home fees (Means and Smith, 1998b; Rummery and Glendinning, 1999).

Commission members were unable to agree unanimously on the best way forward and so it was necessary to publish the main report with a note of dissent signed by two of the members. The main report argued that no logical distinction could be made between health care and social care, and between those services that should be means-tested and those that should be free. This was because:

> Older people need long-term care not simply just because they are old, but because their health has been undermined by a disabling disease such as Alzheimer's Disease, other forms of dementia or a stroke. As yet these diseases cannot effectively be cured by medical care, but people suffering from them will require ongoing therapeutic or personal care of different kinds in order to enable them to live with the disease. In this regard, the only difference between cancer and Alzheimer's Disease is the limitation of medical science. (p 67)

This led the majority of the Commission to conclude that there was a need for a common system for funding personal care that would therefore no longer require a distinction to be made between nursing care and social support (see Figure 2.1). The chosen system was to be free at the point of consumption for service users and paid for through general taxation. Although the public expenditure costs of the proposed changes were considerable (see Table 2.1), the main report argued that they were perfectly affordable.

The two signatories of the note of dissent were not convinced by such arguments. Not only would a reliance on general taxation mean a transfer from the private to the public purse, but "this huge addition to the burden on public expenditure would not, however, increase spending on services for elderly people by a single penny" (p 113). This proved to be the view of the Labour government. It decided that the nursing care element of personal care in nursing homes should become free, but social care in nursing homes, residential care and the community would remain open to means testing and charging. This rejection of the majority view of the Royal Commission was justified on the grounds that "actioning the proposal would absorb huge and increasing sums of money without using any of it to increase the range and quality of care available to older people" (Secretary of State for Health, 2000b).

The government also justified its rejection of the majority view of the

Figure 2.1: Definitions of personal care

Personal care would cover all direct care related to:

- personal toilet (washing, bathing, skincare, personal presentation, dressing and undressing);
- eating and drinking (as opposed to obtaining and preparing food and drink);
- managing urinary and bowel functions (including maintaining continence and managing incontinence);
- managing problems associated with immobility;
- management of prescribed treatment (for example, administration and monitoring medication);
- behaviour management and ensuring personal safety (for example, minimising stress and risk for those with cognitive impairment).

Personal care also includes the associated teaching, enabling, psychological support from a knowledgeable and skilled professional, and assistance with cognitive functions (for example, reminding, for those with dementia) that are needed either to enable a person to do these things for themself or to enable a relative to do them for him/her.

Source: Sutherland Report (1999, p 68)

Table 2.1: Estimated cost of the proposal to exempt personal care from means testing (%)

Year	1995 prices	2010	2021	2031	2051
Cost £ billion	8.2	10.9	14.7	20.8	33.4
Percentage of tax based on earnings + pensions + investments	2.5	2.1	2.1	2.4	2.6
Percentage of GDP	1.2	1.1	1.2	1.3	1.4

Source: Taken from Sutherland Report (1999, p 70, Table 6.8)

Royal Commission on the grounds that it did not fit in with its radical modernisation agenda. The next section focuses on the resultant radical shake up of local authorities in general and social services in particular, and goes on to show how these reforms, together with those associated with the health service, have left open the question of the continuation of the lead agency role of local authorities in community care.

Modernising local authorities and social services

The overall modernisation strategy for local authorities was laid out in *Modern local government: In touch with the people* (Deputy Prime Minister, 1998). This criticised the tendency of local authorities to think in terms of discrete departmental functions rather than from a corporate perspective about how they can benefit citizens irrespective of traditional service boundaries. As a result, the White Paper announced a new duty on local authorities to "promote the economic, environmental and social well-being of their area" (p 10), and this was seen as requiring the forging of partnerships with a wide range of different agencies, including those from the independent sector and the National Health Service.

At the centre of this modernisation agenda for local authorities were two key elements. The first emphasised the need to revitalise local democracy and local governance through such initiatives as elected mayors, local referenda and new political structures (Leach and Wilson, 2000; Rao, 2000). The second was the introduction of 'Best Value' as an alternative to the privatisation of services through compulsory competitive tendering (DETR, 1998).

In terms of Best Value, the 1999 Local Government Act placed a duty on local authorities in England and Wales to "make arrangements to secure continuous improvement in the way (their) functions are exercised, having regard to a combination of economy, efficiency and effectiveness" (Clause 3.1). In addition, this had to be done in such a way that ensured service users and local taxpayers would be empowered to influence and monitor their cost and quality (DETR, 1998, p 6).

Beyond this requirement, Best Value covers a much wider range of services than compulsory competitive tendering (CCT), and expects authorities to consider whether an alternative service provider could provide the service more competitively. This led Geddes and Martin (2000) to claim, "Best Value therefore extends market-like disciplines to the many local authority functions that were not covered by compulsory competitive tendering (CCT) legislation" (p 380). Overall, Best Value reviews have to consider the 'four Cs' (see Figure 2.2), since this is seen as forcing local authorities to establish "demanding targets for efficiency and quality improvements" (DETR, 1998, p 19). A five year programme

Figure 2.2: Best Value and the 'four Cs'

Challenge:	why and how a service is being provided;
Comparison:	with the performance of others across a range of relevant indicators, taking into account the views of both service users and potential suppliers;
Consultation:	with local taxpayers, service users, partners and the wider business community in the setting of new performance targets;
Competition:	as the key means for securing efficient and effective services.

Source: DETR (1999)

of Best Value reviews began in social services in April 2000 and put "everything up for grabs" (Winchester, 2000).

Such general policies on reform in local government have been backed up by more specific modernisation policies for the personal social services. This was justified on the grounds that existing provision and systems had a number of major deficiencies. It was argued that children and vulnerable adults were often not protected, and that services were inflexible and inconsistent across the country while there was "no definition of what users can expect, nor any yardstick for judging how effective or successful social services are" (DoH, 1998a, p 6). Major problems in coordination were also identified:

> Sometimes various agencies put more effort into arguing with one another than into looking after people in need. Frail elderly people can be sent home from hospital, and do not get the support which was promised; or they are forced to stay in hospital while agencies argue about arranging the services they need. (p 5)

The White Paper, *Modernising social services* (DoH, 1998a), argued that the response of Conservative governments had been the privatisation of care provision, which threatened a fragmentation of key services. What was needed was a "third way for social care" which "moves the focus away from who provides the care, and places it firmly on the quality of services experienced by individuals and their carers and families" (p 7).

What was this to mean in practice? The White Paper identified six key reasons why modernisation was essential (see Figure 2.3). In terms of improving protection, it outlined the establishment of a new independent system for protecting vulnerable people, namely a National Care Standards Commission (discussed earlier). With regard to improving standards in the workforce, it announced the creation of a General Social Care Council as well as a variety of other training initiatives. The White Paper also emphasised the need to improve the delivery and efficiency of social services, and this was seen as requiring a renewed emphasis on joint reviews of individual authorities by the Social Services Inspectorate/Audit Commission, the establishment of national priorities guidance (DoH, 1998a, pp 110-12) and a new performance assessment framework (DoH, 1998a, pp 115-17). This was to be combined with the introduction of Best Value reviews for particular aspects of service provision, as already noted.

Figure 2.3: Why modernisation is needed

Protection:	vulnerable children and adults have been exposed to abuse and neglect perpetrated by the very people who were supposed to care for them. Safeguards are not strong enough, and those that are there have not been properly enforced.
Coordination:	older people are left in hospital – so-called 'bedblockers' – while different authorities argue about who should pay for care. The system does not work together well enough to meet people's needs.
Inflexibility:	services sometimes provide what suits the service rather than what the person needs. Just because someone needs care, they do not want their life to be taken over by it – they want the targeted help that they need to get on with their own life, without losing their independence.
Clarity of role:	there is no clear understanding, among the public or the staff, of what services are or should be provided, or what standards can reasonably be expected.
Consistency:	social services cannot be exactly the same everywhere, but a greater degree of consistency is needed. There can be huge differences in standards and levels of service, as well as different systems for deciding who gets what services and how much you might need to pay. All of this leads to a feeling of unfairness.
Inefficiency:	there can be great variation in how much the same services cost in different councils. Social services need to be more efficient, to make sure that the maximum benefit is achieved for the £9 billion of public funding that is spent.

Source: DoH (1998a, pp 5-7)

Finally, as already stressed, *Modernising social services* emphasised the need for improved partnerships, especially in areas such as joint working between health and social services:

> The Government has made it one of its top priorities since coming to office to bring down the "Berlin Wall" that can divide health and social services, and to create a system of integrated care which puts users at the centre of service provision. (p 97)

Joint working was seen as particularly problematic in respect of older people. Services for older people needed to be integrated across health and social care with a greater emphasis upon prevention and rehabilitation so as to reduce the numbers of older people requiring either residential or nursing home care.

Modernising the health services

Aspirations for radical change in health policies were originally outlined in the Green (DoH, 1998b) and White Papers (DoH, 1999) on public health, as well as more generally in the White Paper *The new NHS: Modern, dependable* (DoH, 1997).

The policy documents on public health placed an increased emphasis on the wide environmental determinants of health, yet at the same time stressed that "people can make individual decisions about them and their families' health which can make a difference" (DoH, 1999, p ix). At the centre of this policy was the requirement placed on each health authority to publish a health improvement programme (HIMP) in consultation with key agencies such as social services departments. The content of the HIMP was intended to reflect local needs and priorities, as well as national health targets in priority areas such as cancer, coronary heart disease and stroke, accidents and mental health. These priority areas were also to have their own national service framework and these frameworks were to include one for older people. After some delay, it was finally published in March 2001 (DoH, 2001b).

The new NHS: Modern, dependable emphasised the need for the health service to become primary care rather than hospital driven. It also confirmed the abolition of GP budget holding and its replacement by a new system of primary care groups/primary care trusts based on populations of around 100,000 people. This was seen as involving a four stage developmental process:

Stage One   the primary care group (PCG) acts as an advisory body to its local health authority which retains the health care budget;

Stage Two   the PCG takes devolved responsibility for the budget but remains part of the health authority;

Stage Three   the PCG becomes a primary care trust (PCT) with its own budget and is then a free-standing body accountable to the authority for how it commissions care;

Stage Four   the PCT has added responsibility for providing community services and this is likely to include pooled budgets with social services for much of its community care provision.

Pooled budgets had been made possible by the 1999 Health Act, which swept away a number of past restrictions to joint working. This also made it easier to establish lead commissioning and integrated provider arrangements between health and social services. Finally, the Act had also laid down a more general duty of partnership between health and local authorities on the grounds that:

> People want and deserve the best public services. It is the responsibility of Government, Local Government and the NHS to ensure that those justifiable expectations are met. People care about the quality of a service they get – not how they are delivered or who delivers them. We all need to make sure that service quality does not suffer because of artificial rigidities and barriers within and between service deliverers. (DoH/DETR, 1999)

Indeed, a key feature of government thinking throughout the welfare state modernisation agenda was what the Green Paper on public health called "joined up solutions" (DoH, 1998b, p 12), since need at both the individual and the macro level required responses from a wide range of different professionals and different agencies.

This commitment to the modernisation of the health service was further underlined in July 2000 by the publication of *The NHS plan: A plan for investment, a plan for reform* (Secretary of State for Health, 2000a). As already noted, this announced a massive expansion in training to increase the number of doctors, nurses and professions allied to medicine. It also outlined a series of policy initiatives of direct relevance to older people. This included a £900 million investment by 2003/04 to "build a bridge between hospital and home, by helping people recover and resume independent living more quickly" (p 20). This was seen as not only benefiting the patient but also the hospital in terms of a quicker throughput, so that "by 2004 we will end widespread bed blocking" (p 102). Intermediate care initiatives were expected to include rapid response teams, intensive rehabilitation services, integrated home care teams and social work attachments to primary care.

The NHS Plan also announced a further extension of primary care trusts to levels five and six, going beyond the four stage departmental process outlined above:

> We now propose to establish a new level of primary care trusts which will provide for even closer integration of health and social services. In some parts of the country, health and social services are already working together extremely closely and wish to establish new single multi-purpose legal bodies to commission and be responsible for all local

health and social care. The new body will be known as a 'Care Trust' to
reflect its new broader role. (p 73)

There was also a warning that the government would take powers to
impose care trusts in those localities where inspections and joint reviews
identified a failure to establish effective joint working arrangements.

The NHS Plan also included a chapter specifically on older people.
This made a commitment to establish "a single assessment process for
health and social care" backed up by "a personal care plan" held by the
client/patient (p 125). It confirmed that the National Care Standards
Commission would start its work on driving up standards in domiciliary
and residential care from 2002 and it summarised the response of the
government to the Royal Commission on Long-Term Care (Sutherland
Report, 1999) (discussed earlier).

Understanding the Third Way in public policy

There is a growing amount of literature on what the Labour government
has chosen to call the Third Way in public policy, and the extent to which
it represents an innovative radical new approach rather than a subtle way
of continuing privatisation and the withdrawal of the state in a form
acceptable to most members of the Labour Party (Driver and Martell,
2000; Powell, 1999; Taylor-Gooby, 2000).

The modernisation agenda outlined in this chapter can be presented as
a bold response to the privatisation and quasi-market policies of the
Thatcher and subsequent Conservative governments from 1979 to 1997.
Initial criticisms of a commitment to Conservative spending plans are no
longer relevant and the welfare state has seen a major injection of public
expenditure in recent years. However, not all commentators are convinced.

One option is to conceive the public policies of both Thatcher and
Blair as a response to globalisation pressures. In the late 1970s the Old
Left's belief in a state welfare system funded through taxation came under
attack in most developed economies because of the onset of stagflation
and the end of economic growth combined with a growing fiscal crisis
because of the gap between public expenditure commitments and the
revenue actually being raised (Mishra, 1984). As we have argued elsewhere,
New Right theorists believed that:

> Entrepreneurial energy was being discouraged by excessive taxation
> and excessive regulation. Jobs were not taken up because the
> unemployed were happy to live off social security benefits rather than

take low-paid employment. Finally, the welfare state had become a vast vested interest, largely run for the benefit of those who worked for it. (Means and Smith, 1998b)

The answer was to squeeze state provision to a minimum and to rely wherever possible upon individualism and individual choice. Conservative governments not only supported this but also recognised that competition and market mechanisms could be introduced even where there would never be a fully free market for services (Flynn, 1989). Efficiency was seen as coming from competition and the market.

So how does the modernisation agenda of the Labour government differ from the above, and how does this relate to a different interpretation of globalisation trends? The difference has been well expressed by Driver and Martell (2000):

> So, if New Labour opposes the new Right way, as well as the old Left way, then a third way could promote wealth creation and social justice, the market and the community; it could embrace private enterprise but not automatically favour market solutions; it could endorse a positive role for the state – but need not assume that governments provide public services directly; – and it could, above all, offer a communitarian, rather than individualist view of society in which individuals are embedded in social relations which give structure and meaning to people's lives. (p 149)

The economic argument for such social policies is that a socially integrated society is likely to be an economically successful one, so long as the state is able to produce a highly skilled, motivated and flexible workforce, able to grasp the opportunities offered by information technology and 'e-commerce'. For the less gifted, such an economy would produce numerous opportunities in the lower paid end of the service sector, although IT literacy would often be needed even there.

Therefore, both the state and the individual are seen as crucial because of "the bonding of duties to rights" (Lund, 1999, p 447). The state will help, but only if individuals are willing to help themselves. Not all commentators are convinced of either the fairness or the coherence of this. Taylor-Gooby (2000) has questioned the stress on individual responsibility and has shown how many of those who work in the welfare state believe more emphasis should be placed on tackling structural inequalities and the need for redistributive policies. Powell (2000) argues that behind the rhetoric of modernisation and the Third Way lies only

"PAP: pragmatism and populism", since the reality is so often "policy making on the hoof" in which "what counts is what works".

The confines of this book do not allow for a full exploration of these critiques, other than to comment that Powell seems to give too little credence to the sheer scale of the modernisation policy agenda in health and social care. For example, community care provision for older people is being transformed through the development of care trusts and a host of other initiatives. Clear differences can also be identified between Thatcherism and Blairism over issues such as how to generate efficiency within the welfare state. Conservatives tried to develop market mechanisms by which inefficient providers of health and social care would go out of business if they did not provide what the purchaser/client wanted at a price they could afford. This proved to be an easier approach to take forward when dealing with independent sector social care providers rather than with NHS trusts, and this led the Conservatives to experiment with performance indicators. The modernisation agenda of the Labour government has, from the outset, placed much more emphasis on the need for appraisal and the monitoring of performance as one of the pivots of its whole strategy. National standards, Best Value, clinical governance, evidence based practice, performance frameworks and joint reviews have become the flavour of the day. Central government may believe in markets and competition, but it also believes that its social policy objectives can only be met through the stimulus of extensive surveillance. As such, the Third Way and the modernisation agenda fully embrace what Power (1997) has called the audit society and the rituals of verification.

Modernising community care for older people: key issues with long histories

Although the government has embarked on radical policy change in respect to community care for older people, many of the key issues it faces have long histories as will be illustrated by the rest of this book. These include:

* *Planning versus markets:* governments struggle with how best to 'steer' community care provision for older people. Governments of the early 1970s preferred long-term planning (DHSS, 1972, 1976b, 1977), while the preference of the Conservatives in the 1980s and 1990s was to rely on markets and competition. The subsequent Labour governments, as discussed above, have preferred performance indicators backed up by market incentives.

- *Future of long-term care:* argument and dispute over the respective roles of NHS continuing care beds, residential care and nursing home provision have often dominated debates about health and social care provision for older people to the detriment of concerns about how best to foster their quality of life.
- *Prioritisation and targeting:* one reason for the dominance of the long-term care debate is the public expenditure costs of such provision, and so a third issue has been the level of resources that should be made available for community care provision for older people, and the implications of this for rationing, targeting and prioritisation.
- *The health and social care divide:* the issue of what is health care and what is social care can be traced back to the Poor Law and will feature as a crucial issue in this book as it explores community care provision in the period 1971-93. The Berlin Wall has existed for a long time.
- *Developing the mixed economy:* community care provision for older people has been based on a mixed economy since the Second World War (Means and Smith, 1998a), although the nature of that mixed economy has continued to change and evolve. The emphasis of Conservative governments from 1979 to 1997 was on the need for a contract economy, while the subsequent Labour government extended this further to include the Best Value emphasis on competition, as well as the concept of local compacts between the voluntary sector and local government (Kendall, 2000; Working Group on Government Relations Secretariat/ Local Government Association, 2000). However, all of this has left open to doubt the role of local government as a provider of community care services.
- *What future for social services?* Chapter Seven of this book is very much about social services authorities preparing to take on their role as the lead agency in community care under the 1990 NHS and Community Care Act. However, government proposals on Care Trusts have caused many to doubt whether social services have a key role in the future of community care. A poll of social workers just before the June 2001 general election found that just under three quarters did not expect social services departments to stay in their present form if Labour formed the next government (Downey, 2001).

All of these issues are explored in depth in the next five chapters for the period 1971 to 1993, before the final chapter draws out the policy and practice implications for the modernisation and older people agenda of the present government.

THREE

Targeting, rationing and charging for home care services

Introduction

The previous chapter outlined the modernisation agenda of the present government for the welfare state and its broad implications for services for older people. This chapter begins the process of exploring the roots of some of the issues that need to be tackled by examining the growth of home care services from 1971 to 1993 in the four case study areas (a London Borough, two English Counties and a Metropolitan Authority).

The community care reform elements of the 1990 NHS and Community Care Act were justified by the Conservative government on the grounds that existing provision was service driven, rather than user centred, and that much needed to be done to support people to live in their own homes, rather than allowing them to drift into institutional care (DoH, 1989a, 1990).

Chapter One indicated how this view of the rationale for the community care reforms was completely rejected by some commentators. Sceptical observers saw the changes as a mechanism to cap the public expenditure costs of residential and nursing home care (Hudson, 1990; Lewis and Glennerster, 1996) and to put much greater emphasis on charging and self-provisioning than hitherto. Dominelli and Hoogvelt (1996, p 52) claimed that the 1990 Act brought the market and the contract culture into social work and commented how "social workers are increasingly drawn into becoming managers and accountants, with their time spent pushing paper and pen, or should we say exercising their fingers on the keyboards of their computers, rather than in direct work with users". The community care reforms were seen by many as having undermined a rights-based and free system of care, which was being replaced by an approach driven by the need to ration and to charge, and controlled by managers whose central concern was to stay within budget rather than to meet need. The resultant growth of charging and means testing for domiciliary services since the early 1990s was indeed a major source of anger and frustration for many service users and disability groups (Baldwin and Lunt, 1996; Chetwynd et al, 1996).

This chapter takes a detailed look at home care policy and practice in the period that preceded the 1990 reforms. Was community care provision for older people as bad in the 1970s and 1980s as claimed by the New Right and the market enthusiasts? Do those very critical of the community care changes allow themselves to refer back to a non-existent 'golden age'? The focus is on issues of targeting, rationing and charging for home care, because the apparent consensus by the early 1970s was that older people needed to stay in their own homes for as long as possible, which required intensive home care provision for those most 'at risk' (Means and Smith, 1998a).

Home care prior to 1971

In making this last point it needs to be remembered that governments in the 1940s and 1950s were very reluctant to support the general availability of domiciliary services for older people because of the public expenditure implications (Means and Smith, 1998a, Chapters Four and Six), and this view was often supported by the medical establishment. As late as 1958, Rudd, a consultant physician from a geriatric unit in Southampton, was speaking of how:

> The feeling that the state ought to solve every inconvenient domestic situation is merely another factor in producing a snowball expansion on demands in the National Health (and Welfare) Service. Close observation on domestic strains makes one thing very clear. This is that where an old person has a family who have a sound feeling of moral responsibility, serious problems do not arise, however much difficulty may be met. (Rudd, 1958, pp 348-9)

Other leading geriatricians of the 1950s such as Brooke (1950) and Warren (1951) expressed similar, if less extreme, views.

The primary responsibility for the care of older people was seen as belonging to the family (Means and Smith, 1998a) and this was very much reflected in the 1948 National Assistance Act. As the next chapter shows, the emphasis of this Act was on the reform of public assistance institutions and their replacement with local authority residential homes. The Act did not give local authorities powers to develop what might be called general welfare support for older people who remained in their own homes through the provision of services such as meals on wheels and befriending/visiting schemes. Instead, the 1948 Local Government Act could be used by local authorities to make grants to voluntary organisations so that they could develop such general welfare services (see also Chapter Six). Circular 11/50 on the welfare of old people stressed the urgent need for the voluntary sector to develop these services "which indeed can probably be best provided by voluntary workers actuated by a spirit of good neighbourliness" (MoH, 1950).

Such legislative limitations were harshly criticised. Parker (1965), for example, complained how:

> The concern to maintain and foster family life evident in the Children Act was completely lacking in the National Assistance Act. The latter made no attempt to provide any sort of substitute family life for old people who could no longer be supported by their own relatives. Institutional provision was accepted without question. (p 106)

Legislative change to allow local authorities to develop such services was slow to emerge, despite growing evidence that their availability encouraged families to continue as informal carers (Townsend and Wedderburn, 1965) and that the voluntary sector was unable to develop national coverage (Harris, 1961; Slack, 1960). The 1962 National Assistance (Amendment) Act allowed local authorities to provide meals services directly for the first time, while the 1968 Health Services and Public Health Act provided local authorities with the general power to promote the welfare of older people (implementation of this was delayed until 1 April 1971 and the introduction of the new social services departments).

Throughout this period home care was something of an exception. The modern local authority home help service had its origins in the Second World War when it was introduced initially to support new mothers and then later older people during influenza epidemics. The provision of home help services was confirmed as a discretionary power of local authorities by the 1946 National Health Service Act and it was not until April 1971 that the home help or home care service became a mandatory duty rather than a permissive power.

Despite its discretionary basis, the home help service did show considerable growth in the 1950s and 1960s. The 10 year plans for health and welfare services indicated that in 1961 (MoH, 1963, p 18) 250,000 households were receiving home care because of the needs of a family member who was elderly or chronically ill, and this took up 75% of home help time. However, researchers at the time such as Townsend and Wedderburn (1965), felt that the service was totally inadequate. Many older people in need received no service, many others needed a more intensive service and there were considerable variations in availability between authorities. Such views were supported by research funded by the government, which found that "in order to satisfy the unmet need of present recipients and to provide home help for those who are eligible by present standards but not currently receiving it the size of the home help service would need to be increased by between two and three times a year" (Hunt, 1970, p 25).

In terms of the roots of the home care service it is also important to stress that, despite its consolidation in legislation relating to the health service, it was never seen by civil servants or ministers as being a free service (Lart and Means, 1993). Rather, Aneurin Bevan (Minister of Health) argued in the House of Commons that:

> It is a perfectly reasonable proposition that, where domestic help is needed and the persons concerned are able to provide it for themselves, they should do so, and where they are able to make a contribution they should make it .... It seems to me wholly unjustified that we should provide a service of this sort without any payment whatever. (quoted in Glennerster, 1985, p 147)

The 1946 Act and subsequent circulars gave local authorities wide discretion over their home help charging strategy. For example, section 29 of the Act stated that:

> ... a local authority may, with the approval of the Minister, recover from persons availing themselves of domestic help so provided such charges (if any) as the authority consider reasonable, having regard to the means of those persons.

The implementing circular gave local authorities considerable discretion by giving them freedom:

> ... to determine in each individual case whether any, and if so what charge – within the limits of the standard charge specified in the tariff – would be reasonable, having regard to the means of the person concerned. (quoted in Means and Smith, 1998a, pp 244-5)

In terms of older clients on supplementary pensions, many local authorities agreed arrangements with the local offices of the National Assistance

Table 3.1: Charging policy for home care in the London Borough (1971)[1]

Assessable income (pounds and pence)	Charge per hour (pence)
Up to £16.35	nil
From £16.36 to £16.97	1-10
From £16.98 to £17.24	11-20
From £17.25 to £18.07	21-30
From £18.08 to £18.82	31-39
Over £18.83	40

Board so that the Board would pay a pension supplement to cover the minimum home care charge.

The legislation of the 1940s, therefore, did not provide a rights-based system of home care for older people. The provision of the service was a discretionary power, rather than a mandatory duty. It was seen as a service available to help those older people who lacked strong family support (Means and Smith, 1998a). It was a service where applicants faced a means-tested charge, which local authorities had considerable freedom to set. Many local authorities were not slow to take advantage of this. Central government was sometimes very critical of local authority pricing policies, with one circular claiming that "some of the present arrangements for charges deter people in genuine and even urgent need of the service from taking full advantage of it" (MoH, 1965b).

Towards a right for free home care?

All four case study authorities had a charging policy for the home help service when the new social services authorities came into being in April 1971. The London Borough made no charge for those in receipt of supplementary benefit/pensions from the National Assistance Board. The maximum charge for other clients was 40 pence per hour based on the assessment scale, shown in Table 3.1.

These charges were justified on the grounds that the introduction of a maximum charge for those financially able to pay had the effect of releasing resources for the benefit of people who needed the service but could not afford to pay for it[2].

County Council (B) also had a 40 pence maximum charge, but unlike the London Borough, it also placed a 10 pence per hour charge on those in receipt of supplementary benefit[3]. This arrangement had existed for some time:

> The position in (the County Council) over the last fifteen years has been that by a special arrangement with the (now) Department of Health and Social Security it has been possible to recover 10 pence per hour from recipients of the service who are in receipt of supplementary benefits. In other words a special allowance was made to old people so that they could then pay a contribution towards the cost of providing a home help service for them[4].

It was estimated that this arrangement was generating an income of £30,000 per annum. The other two case studies also charged for home care services with County Council (C) generating an income of £54,000 from client contributions by the mid-1970s, compared with an overall cost of £114,000[5].

However, the early 1970s did witness moves in a direction that was beginning to offer something close to a right to a service. First, local authorities began to place less emphasis on charging for home care in this period. The 1968 Health Services and Public Health Act made the provision of a home help service a mandatory responsibility rather than a discretionary power and this change was implemented on 1 April 1971. It had a major impact on agreements with the National Assistance Board/ Department of Health and Social Security over the payment of supplements to pensioners in receipt of home care. The move to a mandatory duty meant it was no longer appropriate for an eligible person's ability to pay to be dependent on local agreements between local authorities and social security offices. The old approach of dual responsibility was no longer feasible and hence the Director of Social Services (B) felt it necessary to "recommend the Committee to abolish the charge for those in receipt of supplementary benefit"[6], despite the £30,000 per annum loss of income.

In poorer local authorities, this meant that the potential income to be generated through home care charges was now very small indeed. Thus the annual estimates for 1972-73 for the London Borough showed an estimated home care income from charges for 1972-73 of only £6,500[7] and for 1974-75 of only £7,600[8]. The low income figures reflected the fact that out of a home help clientele of 2,057, the great majority, 1,858 (90.3%), were receiving a free service and only 199 (9.6%) were making a financial contribution. Under these circumstances, it was perhaps not surprising that the value of continuing to charge was being questioned in this type of authority:

> ...there are at present three London Boroughs providing a free service....
> The majority of the work involved in assessing this group of paying
> clients is carried out in the Home Help District Offices and it is doubtful
> whether it could be justified on a cost/benefit analysis.... There is a
> natural fear that to make the service 'free' would cause requests to soar,
> but this has not been the experience of the three London Boroughs
> who have made this decision[9].

Soon after this committee discussion, the London Borough abolished its
means-tested home care charging system, as did several other authorities.
The two County Councils, with a significant number of well off older
clients, continued to charge because the income generated justified the
collection expenses, but even in these authorities, the vast majority of
home care recipients were receiving a free service.

In general, the rest of the 1970s and the first half of the 1980s saw
relatively little focus on home care charging issues. This was to change
towards the end of the 1980s as central government began to re-stress the
role of charging and local authorities started to seek ways of income
generation to enable service growth and innovation, despite overall public
expenditure restrictions.

The early 1970s move towards a free service initially coincided with a
period of growth and expansion for the personal social services. During
the late 1960s, the home help service began to expand in response to the
growth in the numbers of older people (Harris, 1968; Hunt, 1970). There
had been virtually no guidance from central government apart from
Circular 25/65, which had merely referred to the importance of assessment
(MoH, 1965b).

Research by Townsend had suggested that home help was mainly offered
to those without support from family and especially female relatives,
although Hunt's survey, published in 1970, painted a rather more complex
picture:

> ...in assessing the amount of help to be given, the majority of organisers
> said they took at least some account of relatives living nearby (although
> many qualified this by saying that the circumstances of the relatives
> would be taken into consideration and no organiser would refuse a
> home help simply because relatives lived nearby). (p 23)

A sympathetic view of the need to support relatives was further encouraged
by Local Authority Circular 53/71. This stressed that the new 1968 Act
referred to households and not individuals, so that "authorities who until

now have felt unable, for example to assist relatives caring single handed for elderly people, may now find advantages in the reconsideration of how to accommodate this need" (DHSS, 1971).

Commentators such as Bosanquet (1978) complained that local authorities continued to place far too much emphasis on the expansion of residential care and this was certainly an important feature of the period (see Chapter Four). However, home care services were expanding in the four case study areas in the early 1970s as part of the general expansion of the personal social services. As one Director of Social Services pointed out, this "meant we had more home helps" (interview with Director of Social Services [A], 1971-80), although the flexibility of what was on offer was usually very limited indeed. Thus, an Assistant Director from the Metropolitan Authority spoke of a pattern in which "you can have whatever home help you need as long as it's three hours a week in the morning" (interview with Assistant Director of Social Services [D], 1977-87).

Nevertheless, this was a period of great optimism when it was expected that budgets would roll on in the following year with an addition that would be greater than inflation. Central government was asking local authorities to submit 10 year plans based on an increase of 10% each year in real terms (DHSS, 1972). Incremental growth was the expected norm and one that was perhaps turning access to a basic home help service into an expectation (and almost a right) for those older people who turned to social services for support additional to that which was available from their families.

From boom to bust

In his study of the welfare state in Britain since 1945, Lowe (1999) stressed how developments in welfare are influenced by a range of factors that include both economic and political considerations. Community care commentators have tended to emphasise political factors and more specifically the impact of the ideology of Thatcherism on changing policy and practice within the personal social services. However, a close study of the four case studies shows that it is equally important to stress the economic factors that preceded the arrival of a Conservative government in 1979. Drawing on Lowe, Table 3.2 underlines the importance of this and shows how periods of economic crisis within the stop-go cycle of the period included the early to mid-1970s. This period also saw a massive rise in inflation, reaching 16.1% in 1973-74 and 23.1% in 1974-75. The honeymoon period for social services authorities was at an end. The

1975 annual conference of Directors of Social Services had presentations on 'manpower planning and training in a no growth situation', 'voluntary organisations in a time of financial crisis' and 'the organisation of social services departments in a time of limited resources'[10].

The impact on the four case study authorities was considerable. Social Services Committee (D) received a paper on 26 August 1975 from the Management Board of the local authority on "The effects on the corporate plan of government action to attack inflation"[11]. This was a response to the government paper, *The attack on inflation* (HM Government, 1976), which had seen reductions in public expenditure and the public sector borrowing requirement as critical to the achievement of this aim. The Management Board paper warned that "present indications however are that a stop in non-committed growth will not be sufficient to meet the Government's requirements"[12]. The emphasis had switched to "priorities for maintaining present activities rather than options for growth"[13]. A subsequent paper called specifically for "a reduction in 1976/77 expenditure of 7% from the existing level"[14].

The Social Services Committee of County Council (C) was looking for savings of £110,000 for 1977-78[15]. The members of the Social Services Committee of the other County Council (B) were being told by their

Table 3.2: Major stimuli to economic expansion and contraction (1969-74)

	'Stop'	'Go'
1969 April	Budget – £340m	
1971 March		Budget + £256m
1972 April		Budget + £1,211m
		Barber boom
1972 July		£ floated
1973 October	OPEC oil price rises	
1973 December	Public expenditure cuts	
1974 February		Social Contract
1974 March		Healey budget

Notes: unbroken lines denote a change of government, dotted lines peaks of the economic cycle. Figures for the budget specify the extent to which *The Economist* estimated it expanded or contracted the economy. Anthony Barber and Denis Healey were Chancellors of the Exchequer in 1972 and 1974 respectively.
Source: Taken from Lowe (1999, p 71)

Director that "we are now in a period of the most severe restrictions on public expenditure and no improvement to standards of service can reasonably be expected for a minimum of five years"[16], while a very similar message was being delivered to members in the London Borough[17].

However, the outcome of such deliberation in most local authorities was not a dramatic review of who should be entitled to home care. The reason for this was the advice laid out clearly in the government Circular on *Local authority expenditure in 1976/77 – forward planning* (DHSS, 1975). This stated: "the Government's view is that authorities should not reduce the effectiveness of the field and domiciliary services or curtail the urgent expansion of specialist residential provision for children", (see also DHSS, 1976b, pp 38-41). Instead, local authorities were advised to delay other new capital works, reduce the numbers for whom residential care was being planned and reduce "expenditure on services that are provided generally, without regard to individual need and on long term preventative activities".

The four case studies took a variety of strategies to achieve their cutback targets. Thus, the London Borough gave capital schemes a rank order and made estimates of likely capital and revenue savings[18], but later went on to question the value of some of its more general preventative schemes for older people, such as drop in luncheon clubs, holidays and Christmas cards[19]. The Social Services Committee of County Council (B) was asked to note how "the capital building programme had been virtually abandoned"[20] already because of the need to switch resources to domiciliary services and was therefore asked to accept that the only way to make further savings in services for older people was through targeting help at the following groups:

- those people aged over 75 and living alone where the withholding of services would inevitably mean their needing admission to hospital or an old people's home in the short term;
- those old people discharged from hospital where family or neighbour support was not available or needed to be supplemented[21].

The inevitable consequence of this shift was seen to be that County Council (B) would be "dealing predominantly with crisis situations rather than concentrating on preventative support"[22].

County Council (C) also went down the route of delaying and reducing previously agreed capital projects, including not opening three new schemes (a day centre, a hostel for people with learning difficulties and a residential home for older people) in order to make revenue savings and stay within overall staffing targets for social services[23]. The Metropolitan Authority also concentrated upon the need to reduce capital programmes with the Social Services Committee being asked "to have regard to the effect of any such schemes on their revenue budgets for subsequent years"[24].

Despite the 'stop-go' economic cycles of the period, governments were becoming convinced that the kind of broad welfare service growth for older people associated with the early 1970s could not be sustained in the future, even with a significant economic upturn. This message was rammed home by *A happier old age* (DHSS, 1978a), the consultative paper produced by the Labour government a year before the election of the first Thatcher administration. The picture presented by this document was *not* of a welfare system that could provide domiciliary and other welfare services as a right and free of charge. Instead, the context was one of a rising overall older population, combined with significant increases in the numbers of the 'old old'. The paper pointed out "that roughly speaking just over £10,000 million, or a third of the total public expenditure on the main social programmes, is attributable to elderly people" and that "within the health and personal social services the average cost of care and treatment of a person aged over 75 is seven times that of a person of working age" (p 10).

The policy implications of this situation for welfare services were clearly laid out in the paper. There needed to be reduced reliance on residential care through the more effective use of community-based health and welfare services. However, this required a much clearer approach to targeting for services such as home care than in the past because of public expenditure restrictions:

> Development of the domiciliary services has so far largely relied on professional judgements and been influenced by demands pressed against a background of growth in the national economy and rising expectations.... However, it is vital to make the best use of all available resources, to deploy these in a way which gives elderly people – and their relatives – the kind of help they need, and to ensure that those in greatest need are given priority. (p 33)

In the 1980s, this was often interpreted to mean that those older people at risk of residential care needed access to appropriate home support in order to avoid admission to care.

Towards the targeting of home care services?

The kind of policy framework suggested by *A happier old age*, was reinforced strongly with the arrival of a Conservative government in 1979. Both its White Paper on *Growing older* (DHSS, 1981c) and the handbook on *Care in action* (DHSS, 1981a) stressed that "care in the community must increasingly mean by the community" (DHSS, 1981c, p 3) because "public authorities will not command the resources to deal with it alone" (DHSS, 1981a, p 32). In other words, the provision of home care services could only be justified when targeted at those most likely to end in residential care despite informal support.

This encouraged searching questions to be asked of the effectiveness of existing home care services. As early as 1977, a study by Plank (1978) had suggested that the amount of home care available to individual clients was insufficient to prevent the admission to residential care of those older people judged by social workers to be capable of independent living. As Davies (1981) argued in the early 1980s:

> The service generally shows too even a distribution among recipients who vary greatly in their need for help.... Only in relatively few areas is home help available at weekends and out of office hours to those truly on the crucial margins of need for residential care. It seems that in few areas has the budget been used to provide resources for personal rather than domestic care. (p 50)

Goldberg and Connelly (1982) in a review of the literature argued that "one of the most important general issues implicit in a number of studies is how to arrive at the 'right' balance between meeting the more general needs of the elderly population for domiciliary support and giving intensive services to those most 'at risk' who wish to stay in their own homes" (p 80).

The push from government continued to emphasise the need for an intensive service for the few (Audit Commission, 1985; Social Services Inspectorate, 1987, 1988) in which home care staff would be expected to take on a growing amount of personal care tasks. Sinclair and Williams (1990) outlined a nationally negotiated job description that seemed to reflect these changes:

> The duties will include domestic tasks (including cleaning, cooking and washing), physical tasks approximating to home care (including dressing, washing and feeding clients), and social duties (including talking

with clients, helping clients to maintain contact with family, friends and community, assisting with shopping and recreation), aimed at creating a supportive, homely atmosphere where clients can achieve maximum independence. (p 164)

They pointed out that numerous local authorities had changed the name of the service, from home help to home care, to reflect this growing emphasis on intensive personal care for highly dependent older people.

So how did the four case studies respond to these kinds of pressures? The London Borough had decided on the need for a "wide-ranging review of policies and practices" in relation to services for older people in June 1981[25]. At this time, the recently arrived Director of Social Services was very keen "to reduce the dependence on residential care for older people" and "to increase and improve the strength and the quality of our domiciliary support services" (interview with Director of Social Services [A], 1980-83). More specifically, services were reorganised in order to facilitate a move from a "home help and cleaning service" to a home care or "personal care service" (interview with Director of Social Services [A], 1980-83).

The result of such deliberations was the establishment in 1984 of priority categories (see Figure 3.1), which distinguished between the characteristics of those clients requiring help seven days per week and those that would be considered if resources allowed[26]. These categories were still in operation six years later, but had come under increasing pressure because of a recruitment freeze:

> Currently, there are now 28 FTE vacancies. This explains the increase in the number of unallocated cases to 296 in June/August 1990 and, in addition, a number of allocated cases will only be receiving a reduced service either on a regular basis, or ad hoc basis; for example, it may not be possible to cover when a home help is off sick. A number of the lowest category clients (categories I and J, normal service one day per week) have received no service over the Summer and this position is likely to continue until the New Year[27].

These comments suggest the traditional rationing methods of waiting lists and reduced service (Lart and Means, 1993) were being used as much as, and possibly more than, the targeting of services to those deemed most in need. By 1990, the pressure to review the situation was becoming intense because of the need to offer more support to carers and to develop

Figure 3.1: Priorities for home helps (London Borough)

Clients in categories A-C need seven days per week help

A   Clients who are assessed as being highly vulnerable, through physical frailty or confusion, in that they need assistance with getting up in the morning; dressing; washing; provision of breakfast; assistance to eat; provision of a late meal; considerable assistance with budgeting, and so on, in order to remain at home. Likely to need three visits per day.

B   Clients who are highly vulnerable from physical frailty, in that they need assistance to get up in the morning, wash and dress, but who can feed themselves if food is prepared for them, because of infirmity cannot attend day facilities. Likely to need two visits per day at breakfast and teatime.

C   Clients who are highly vulnerable through physical frailty, in that they need assistance to dress, assistance to prepare a meal, but have very restricted mobility around the house, although they are not able to go to day centres, and so on. Likely to need one visit per day.

D   Clients who are highly vulnerable in that they need assistance to dress and prepare a meal, but who are able to be cared for at a day facility or by a relative. Likely to need one visit per week.

E   Clients who are highly vulnerable, but have assistance from relatives, friends and volunteers available during the week or at weekends. Need help five days per week, only for assistance to get up, dress and feed.

Clients in categories F-J will be considered if space allows

F   Clients with a physical disability who need assistance with cleaning, laundry, shopping (collecting of pension) and occasional preparation of meals, emptying commode, and so on.

G   Clients with a physical disability who need help with heavy shopping and cleaning or laundry. Clients mobile indoors, but living in difficult accommodation (for example, stairs to flat), which hinder their going out.

H   Clients with a physical disability who can carry out many tasks within the home, (for example, cleaning, cooking), but who are unable to go out and need assistance with shopping and laundry.

I   Clients who are vulnerable through frailty, who can undertake the majority of household tasks, but need assistance with heavy cleaning and shopping and need prompting to encourage their independence. Problems will arise if help is not given, as the client is likely to require more help in the long-term.

J   Clients who are vulnerable, who need a visit only occasionally (fortnightly) for heavy cleaning tasks

"an evening and extended week-end service for those with severest need"[28].

At quite an early stage, County Council (B) recognised that its very large older population meant that it was not feasible to meet needs through local authority residential care. Even in the mid-1970s, the emphasis was not only on making use of the private and voluntary sector residential provision[29], but also on switching resources from the capital programme to concentrate efforts on "sustaining people in their own homes by developing the domiciliary and community services"[30]. It has already been noted that this Council introduced eligibility criteria about who could be helped, with an emphasis on old people living alone and hospital discharge situations. However, a 1979 survey found that although a significant number of clients were receiving personal care as well as more basic support, "few of the elderly had very severe handicaps though a significant percentage had appreciable or minor ones"[31].

The need to improve this state of affairs continued to be recognised throughout the 1980s, although with little apparent change in the overall situation. In 1984, the Social Services Committee was told of the need for the home care service to broaden its scope by "extending its role further in the community ... by further hospital discharge schemes, night sleeping or sitting services and further liaison with community nursing and voluntary schemes"[32].

However, it was proving difficult to find the resources to set up enhanced services. Four years later a strategy report complained that:

> The additional funding in 1987/88 assisted in keeping pace with demographic trends and the more quantifiable increase in demands being placed upon the Department. £32,000 was required in 1988/89 to keep pace with these changes. This failed to materialise and consequently the service was reduced in real terms, against the back-drop of an already minimal service compared with stated committee policy[33].

In the late 1980s, County Council (B) carried out consumer research on both domiciliary services and residential care. These studies found that the home care service in particular was seen as popular and effective, but that the public had inadequate knowledge of the full range of services that might be offered (night sitter services, respite care, and so on). They also found that:

> Research into admissions to residential care revealed that half of all those admitted would have preferred to have stayed in their own homes and a half of those could have been supported in their own homes with reasonable levels of domiciliary services[34].

It should be remembered that the Council had set this as a goal right from the early days of the social services department.

County Council (C) was initially much more cautious than County Council (B) about abandoning its traditional reliance on local authority residential homes. One option being considered in June 1981 was the closure of a home with high maintenance costs and in need of refurbishment. A report to the Social Services Committee pointed out:

> ... some authorities are taking opportunities to develop alternative provision because these are said to maintain people in their own homes and/or cost less. Such schemes, which would still have to be evaluated in terms of need, practicability and demographic change as far as Case Study C is concerned, include:
>
> a) extended domiciliary care services;
> b) foster care for the elderly;
> c) use of agency accommodation;
> d) joint assessment schemes with health authorities;
> e) rationalised use of existing accommodation[35].

However, the thrust of the report was not one of ringing endorsement for such change since it stressed that "it is essential, if any of these courses are to be considered, that further studies are made and reports presented before a final decision is made"[36].

This local authority continued to look at residential versus domiciliary care options for older people throughout the early 1980s. In particular it looked at the findings from a joint finance project in one part of the county that had examined the possibility of maintaining older people in their own homes by the provision of enhanced domiciliary support beyond the point at which they would otherwise be admitted to institutional care. The conclusion was that this did work, but only under certain circumstances. Home care staff needed additional training and the full support of health care agencies was required[37]. It remained true that "there are clearly some cases where, because of the client's high dependence level, the extent of required project services is not cost-effective"[38]. The crunch issue in any authority-wide expansion of the scheme was seen as the need for clear criteria that could identify those for whom the scheme would be cost effective.

County Council (C) did continue to experiment with a variety of approaches to the delivery of home care services, including the use of rapid response teams[39] and a growing emphasis on the need for tighter targeting. Indeed more explicit eligibility criteria were introduced in 1987, and further refined in 1991, and these emphasised the need to take into consideration (a) dependency level, (b) support available to the client and (c) the risk factor of not providing a service[40]. The emphasis was on switching to meeting the needs of those "requiring high inputs of care which may require a care assistant visiting up to three times a day"[41]. The end result was a switch to a more intensive service for a small number of clients:

> The number of clients receiving home care has reduced over the last 12 months from 4,955 to 4,200. This is partly due to the charging system, and partly because the average number of hours per client has increased from 3.60 to 3.87[42].

Nevertheless, the Director of Social Services remained dissatisfied with the overall situation. A disproportionate percentage of the social services budget continued to be spent on local authority residential care (see Chapter Four), so that "large numbers of elderly people do not receive a service at all"[43]. Financial difficulties within the local authority meant that planned growth in community services could not take place in 1991–92, leaving the Director to express concern at "how little of the strategy has been implemented"[44].

The Metropolitan Authority was also quite slow to consider if it should begin to offer a more intensive service for a smaller number of clients. The main policy statement and options report for the period 1980-83 for social services outlined how 3,537 clients were receiving 10,863 hours of home help. It also explained how the "service provides practical support to people in their own homes, who could not otherwise maintain themselves" and that "the service is available to a wide range of clients although 90% of home help recipients are elderly and the majority of these are in the 75+ age group"[45].

However, a major reconsideration of this situation took place in the mid-1980s as a result of reviews of services for older people in 1982 and the home help service in 1983[46]. The first report stressed how the growth of residential care places had not kept pace with the older population, so that many more of the heavily dependent were staying in the community with domiciliary care support. The second had stressed "that a significant proportion of clients required substantial assistance with 'personal care' tasks such as dressing, washing, toileting and meal preparation"[47]. The proposed way forward was the establishment of 20 additional home help posts to help the service further embrace personal care tasks as well as household duties, with the priority being the provision "of intensive and flexible support in the home to elderly people who are physically or mentally frail"[48]. In line with this, the policy statement and options paper for 1987-90 referred to the home care rather than home help service, and stated that in recent years the service had "been expected to provide an increasingly intensive and flexible response to the needs of the growing numbers of dependent elderly people in the community"[49].

The authority continued to push this approach further. The transfer of a residential home to a housing association was used to help further expand the home care service as part of a commitment to change the balance of care, between care in the community and care in residential homes[50]. However, "changes in health service provision (shorter in-patient care, more out-patient treatment, fewer hospital beds)"[51], combined with demographic change, were seen as undermining the ability to achieve this shift. As a result, a 1988 report to the Social Services Committee continued to describe this as a service that "basically operates in normal working hours"[52].

Nevertheless, pressure for change continued to build up. The local authority had an over provision of residential places with resultant high vacancy rates in some homes, while the need to bring local authority homes up to the same registrable standard as independent sector homes for April 1991, created a massive capital investment dilemma[53]. In the end, two homes were closed and eight were transferred to an independent organisation (see Chapter Four). The resultant savings were invested in home care services, so that by late 1991 a report to the Social Services Committee felt able to claim that "the pattern of provision of services for elderly people is changing rapidly as the Home Care Service develops a more comprehensive range of care, covering not just weekdays but weekends and in the evening and night"[54].

Overall, the picture is of all four case study authorities moving in the direction of more targeted home care services, but in a situation where they were continuing to face difficulties in turning these policies into reality on the ground. In interviews, senior managers from these social services departments were very honest about two of the main reasons for this. First, when financial cuts are faced it is often a case of "children before everything" and in terms of adult services "you cut home care because it's hard to close old people's homes" (interview with Director of Social Services [C], 1988-95). Or, as another interviewee put it, when "you're going to overspend it was always the poor old home help services that in fact we cut back" (interview with Senior Manager, roles included County Advisor for Elderly People [C], 1971-89). As a result, aspirations to develop evening and weekend cover were often delayed. Second, the previous practices of home help staff needed to be changed, and this was often a long and sometimes expensive process. It required retraining, negotiations with trades unions and often changed contracts of employment. The outcome was often a more expensive service, so that by the early 1990s in County Council (C) "improved pay and conditions for home care assistants, including guaranteed hours of work and salaried status, have been introduced as the essential basis for flexible coverage of intensive personal care needs, often at unsocial hours, leading to increased cost of service per hour"[55]. The end result was often slow progress, which is compatible with the findings from the literature review by Sinclair and Williams (1990), which identified "an overall lack of change in the intensity with which home help is provided" (p 165).

Conclusion

Many commentators have associated the Griffiths Report (1988), the White Paper on community care (DoH, 1989a) and the 1990 NHS and Community Care Act as ushering in an emphasis on charging, rationing and the narrow targeting of home care services for older people. This chapter has presented a rather different and more complex picture, in which the roots of such policies and practices can be traced back well before these policy developments. There has never been a period in which all local authorities provided universally available free home care, although the importance of charges as a mechanism for part funding the service did decline in the 1970s and 1980s (Sinclair and Williams, 1990), only to revive in the early 1990s (Lart and Means, 1993). The home help service did expand in the early 1970s and for a time in the mid to late 1970s it was protected from review in most local authorities by the 'slack' in the capital building programme. But pressure to review the objectives of the service and to focus on how it could contribute to keeping people out of residential care was a source of major debate at both the national and local levels for at least 10 years before the publication of the Griffiths Report (1988). However, it can be argued that this was much more at the level of rhetoric and local political debate, rather than in terms of sustained change on the ground.

Notes

[1] Social Services Committee (A), 25 October 1971 (Review of Charges).

[2] Ibid.

[3] Social Services Committee (B), 8 December 1971 (The Home Help Service).

[4] Ibid.

[5] Social Services Committee (C), 10 September 1976 (1976/77 Budget).

[6] Social Services Committee (B), 8 December 1971 (The Home Help Service).

[7] Social Services Committee (A), 25 October 1971 (Review of Charges).

[8] Social Services Committee (A), 25 November 1974 (Review of Charges).

[9] Ibid.

[10] Report of Proceedings of the Social Services Conference, 1975 (AMA: London and ACC: London).

[11] Social Services Committee (D), 26 August 1975 (The Effects on the Corporate Plan of Government Action to Attack Inflation).

[12] Ibid.

[13] Ibid.

[14] Social Services Committee (D), 15 January 1976 (Budget, 1976/77).

[15] Social Services Committee (C), 28 May 1976 (Budget Plans, Manpower Planning and the Public Expenditure White Paper).

[16] Social Services Committee (B), 2 September 1975 (Priorities for the Social Services Department).

[17] Social Services Committee (A), 27 October 1975 (Local Authority Expenditure in 1976/77 – Forward Planning).

[18] Social Services Committee (A), 3 September 1975 (Future Levels of Council Expenditure).

[19] Social Services Committee (A), 3 September 1975 (References from the Elderly, Physically Handicapped and Ill and Community Development Review Committee).

[20] Social Services Committee (B), 2 September 1975 (Priorities for the Social Services Department).

[21] Ibid.

[22] Ibid.

[23] Social Services Committee (C), 28 May 1976 (Budget Plans, Manpower Planning and the Public Expenditure White Paper).

[24] Social Services Committee (D), 25 January 1977 (Policy Options, 1977-78).

[25] Social Services Committee (A), 16 June 1981 (Social Services Budget and Forward Programme, 1981-82).

[26] Social Services Committee (A), 22 October 1990 (Domiciliary Services Review).

[27] Ibid.

[28] Ibid.

[29] Social Services Committee (B), 30 September 1974 (Position Statement: Social Services).

[30] Social Services Committee (B), 2 September 1975 (Priorities for the Social Services).

[31] Social Services Committee (B), 21 June 1979 (Services for the Elderly).

[32] Social Services Committee (B), 21 June 1984 (Statement of General Strategy: Services for the Elderly).

[33] Social Services Committee (B), 23 June 1988 (Social Services Strategy to 1990 – Monitoring and Review, 1988).

[34] Social Services Committee (B), 15 September 1989 (Review of Domiciliary Services).

[35] Social Services Committee (C), 13 June 1981 (Closure of an Old People's Home).

[36] Ibid.

[37] Social Services Committee (C), 11 September 1981 (Alternative Placements).

[38] Social Services Committee (C), 3 December 1982 (Residential versus Domiciliary Care for the Elderly).

[39] Social Services Committee (C), 8 March 1989 (Quarterly Financial Report).

[40] Social Services Committee (C), 20 May 1991 (Domiciliary Care – Service and Budget Review).

[41] Ibid.

[42] Social Services Committee (C), 10 September 1991 (Home Care Charges).

[43] Social Services Committee (C), 10 December 1991 (Services for Elderly People).

[44] Ibid.

[45] Social Services Committee (D), 22 January 1980 (Policy Statement and Options 1980–83).

[46] Social Services Committee (D), 24 September 1985 (Domiciliary Services for Elderly People).

[47] Ibid.

[48] Ibid.

[49] Social Services Committee (D), 14 December 1987 (Policy Statement and Options, 1987-90).

[50] Social Services Committee (D), 24 January 1989 (Corporate Plan and Budget, 1989-90).

[51] Social Services Committee (D), 22 November 1988 (Financial Planning Total, 1989-90).

[52] Social Services Committee (D), 27 September 1988 (Policy Statement 1988).

[53] Social Services Committee (D), 22 November 1990 (Development of Services for Elderly People).

[54] Social Services Committee (D), 17 September 1991 (Policy Statement).

[55] Social Services Committee (C), 20 May 1991 (Domiciliary Care: Service and Budget Review).

FOUR

The changing role of local authority residential care

Introduction

The focus of this chapter is on the changing nature of local authority residential care from 1971 to 1993 in terms of such issues as capital investment, the level of dependency of residents, the impact of market competition and the growing emphasis on consumer rights.

Our previous research explored the role of such care in the earlier period from the outbreak of the Second World War through to the creation of social services departments in April 1971 (Means and Smith, 1998a). The study focused on how the 1948 National Assistance Act attempted to replace the old public assistance institution with a new form of non-stigmatising residential home to be run by local authorities:

> The old institutions are to go altogether. In their place will be attractive hostels or hotels, each accommodating 25 to 30 old people, who will live there as guests not inmates. Each guest will pay for his accommodation – those with private income out of that, those without private income out of the payments they get from the National Assistance Board – and nobody need know whether they have private means or not. Thus, the stigma of 'relief' – very real too, and acutely felt by many old people – will vanish at last. (Public Assistance Officer, quoted in Means and Smith, 1998a, p 155)

Yet the expected new homes were not built in the 1950s because of general restrictions on capital investment programmes during the post-war period of austerity and because older people were seen as a low priority for whatever capital was available.

Local authorities coped with this situation in two main ways. First, they continued to make extensive use of former public assistance institutions. A Ministry of Health (1959) report suggested many of these buildings had been updated (large dormitories partitioned, ceilings lowered, new heating systems installed, floors carpeted, and so on) but that "nevertheless there are still former institutions which have shown little change since 1948" (p 239). Second, large existing homes were bought, often "in splendid grounds, offloaded onto the market by the erstwhile wealthy, left servantless and impoverished by the war" (Kemp, 1973, p 496). Such homes were often in luxurious surroundings, but tended to be in very isolated positions and with very limited access for disabled people.

The inadequacy of the overall situation was vividly exposed by the detailed research on residential care carried out by Townsend (1962) and published in *The last refuge*. This attacked not only the poor quality of residential home buildings, but also the poor quality of many residential care staff. A particular concern was with those who had trained under the Poor Law. Townsend argued that "it would be idle to pretend that many of them were imbued with the more progressive standards of personal care encouraged by the Ministry of Health and that a minority were unsuitable, by any standards, for the tasks they performed, men or women with authoritarian attitudes inherited from Poor Law days who provoked resentment and even terror among infirm people" (p 39).

Townsend's broad conclusion was that all long stay institutions failed to give residents "the advantages of living in a 'normal' community" (p 190), and hence should be abandoned as an instrument of social policy. He argued that most older residents could live in the community with improved pensions, better housing (including sheltered housing) and with support from domiciliary services. The response by central government was to focus more on the need to replace out of date buildings with modern purpose-built residential homes. This was based on the belief that such care was cheaper than geriatric care in the NHS. The late 1960s saw an extensive capital investment in the building of new residential homes for older people (Means and Smith, 1998a, Chapter Five).

Large-scale production of new homes in a land of plenty?

The previous chapter outlined how the early 1970s was a period of substantial growth in the provision of public services (Lowe, 1999) and this trend was strongly reflected in the personal social services in general and in provision for older people in particular (Means et al, 2000). One consequence of this was a period of further rapid growth in the development of new local authority residential care homes.

Thus a progress report on capital works for the London Borough in

October 1972 identified one old people's home as completed, one under construction and another as an agreed new project[1]. County Council (B) had estimated that they would need £2,580,117 for capital projects for "residential accommodation for the aged" in the period 1971/72 to 1974/75[2]. County Council (C) had also developed an extensive capital programme (£8,615,570 by 1977/78) with the same emphasis on new build residential care for older people[3]. The Metropolitan Authority was also concerned with the need for new homes[4] and its then Director of Social Services stated that "expenditure for the early period was more of the same", especially where this involved "new shiny residential homes" (interview with Director of Social Services [D], 1971-87).

At times senior managers seemed to be in the luxurious position of being able to identify preferred sites and sizes of residential homes for different communities. This is vividly illustrated by three quotations from County Council (B):

> I was saying [the Deputy Director] and I spent an evening in County Hall with a map of the County where we mapped out together with projected population figures, the building programme where we put in the larger towns a 50 bedded home, a 40 bedded home in the smaller ones and in the very small ones there would be 15 bedded homes. (interview with Senior Services Manager [B], 1971-90 [Director of Social Services from 1985-90])

> When I look back at the times in the middle sixties, you know we were having a 10 per cent growth, can you imagine? We were building 15 bedded homes in small towns.... I was very concerned about size, so we were looking at unit homes in the bigger homes, you know, dividing a 50 bedded home.... And we had money, you know. And we were pretty free because the government grants depended on the number of old people you had and the length of roads, and its funding was altered. And (B) was a very rural county, so we wanted to produce local services so that old people who hadn't left in the whole of their lives wouldn't spend the last three or four years of their life 50 miles away. (interview with Senior Social Services Manager [B], 1971-90)

> I can remember one of the first jobs that I had to do. It was a sort of wish list really of development of services across the board. One of the first jobs I had to do was to look at the possible siting throughout (B) of new old people's homes. We went through the population levels of the County looking at the largest towns which didn't have an old

people's home, and it was that crude, you know. But that just describes
… people's expectations and hope for the development of the service,
because at that time it was a real boom industry. And budgets were
going up a significant amount every year … it was a great time because
… individual wishes almost came true. (interview with Registration
and Inspection Officer [B], 1971-87)

Commentators from that period (Bosanquet, 1978) and more recent
authors (Means and Smith, 1998b) have been very critical of this emphasis
on investment in residential care rather than domiciliary and other home-
based support services. However, social services authorities had inherited
from welfare departments some properties in desperate need of either
closure or a massive overhaul. These were a mixture of the last few
former public assistance institutions still in use, as well as many of the
older converted properties bought in the 1950s and early 1960s. Thus in
the London Borough, the social services authority was struggling with
the following residential home for older people:

… one very large room on the ground floor has been divided into two.
Six gentlemen sleep in one half, seven gentlemen in the other. The
ceiling is high; adding to the institutional feeling of the room, but the
main cause for concern is the overcrowding and subsequent lack of any
possibility of privacy. The beds have to be set side by side and are separated
by a space of less than three feet, that space being taken up by a locker[5].

Such homes were often used for older men or women who had led an
itinerant lifestyle and hence who were expected to object less to the lack
of privacy and personal space associated with such out of date facilities.
In a similar vein, the Social Services Committee of County Council
(C) was told in December 1971 of the need for a review of appropriate
standards of buildings and facilities in residential homes for older people,
since "some accommodation will have to be vacated because it falls below
standards, others will need to be adapted and improved"[6]. As late as 1982,
County Council (B) still had 14 rooms in eight homes where more than
three older people slept together[7].

Whatever the reason for this emphasis on capital investment for new
residential care homes, it has already been shown that this was not a
period that lasted for long. The oil and sterling crises of the mid-1970s,
combined with high inflation, meant that the days of 10% annual growth
in real terms and large capital programmes could not be sustained. Priority
guidance from the government was clear that the emphasis should be

towards domiciliary services rather than residential care as in the past because of "the expense of these facilities in relation to the domiciliary services" (DHSS, 1976b, p 42). Indeed the easiest way for local authorities to cope with the severe public expenditure cutbacks of the period was to reduce capital programmes with the resultant knock-on consequences of reduced future revenue costs (an unopened home does not need to be staffed). Typical was the Metropolitan Authority in January 1977 when members were asked to reduce capital programmes and "to have regard to the effect of any such schemes on their revenue budgets for subsequent years"[8], while 15 months earlier County Council (B) members had been asked to note that "the capital building programme has been virtually abandoned"[9].

The previous chapter demonstrated how one consequence of all this was a growing emphasis on the need to develop domiciliary services that could enable dependent older people to avoid residential care. However, despite this rhetoric, social services departments of the period continued to spend an enormous amount of time and energy on issues related to local authority residential homes. This chapter explores two reasons for this. The first was the increased dependency and ill health of those who remained in residential care and the second related to the spectacular growth of independent sector residential and nursing home care in the mid-1980s.

It is important to appreciate that such restrictions on capital expenditure did not only affect prospects for the building of new purpose-built homes. It also impacted on proposals for the maintenance and updating of existing homes.

The cost of updating even one home could be considerable, as illustrated by the following example from the Metropolitan Authority:

> This home does not readily adapt to a group living arrangement but could be significantly improved by the following alterations:
>
> a) extension and alterations to the lounges;
> b) additional WCs and Parker bath;
> c) new lift;
> d) additional storage and alterations to the laundry;
> e) provision of ramped access;
> f) alterations to the staff accommodation.
>
> The Director of Development and Town Planning has prepared an indicative estimate of the cost which is £96,000[10].

The cost of this updating was seen as problematic and so the six month waiting time for the delivery of the lift was seen as having the advantage of spreading the cost over two financial years.

However, even much smaller scale upgrades could soon generate significant potential expenditure. Thus, the proposed capital programme for 1981/82 in County Council (B) included 21 improvements for 14 different local authority residential homes, with works ranging from 'tap and hose in dustbin area' at a cost of £150 to a general conversion of toilets and bathrooms to accommodate wheelchair access that was going to cost £18,100. Other required improvements included 'handrails to steps leading to a garden' (£1,200), conversion of a double bedroom into a day care room (£3,500) and the introduction of a call bell system (£6,000)[11]. Under these circumstances, even routine maintenance such as external painting and internal redecoration was always likely to be pared back to a minimum[12, 13, 14, 15], with County Council (C) considering the increased use of residential home staff to carry out these functions[16].

Because of the growing restrictions on public expenditure, local authorities had to deal with the tension between updating/upgrading and carrying out routine maintenance. The pressure to upgrade came from the growing dependency levels of residents (see next section), but overall what was happening, as will be seen later in this chapter, was an enormous backlog of demand for both general repairs/maintenance and major improvements.

The challenge of increasing dependency

Our previous research illustrated how "in need of care and attention" was redefined on several occasions during the 1950s and 1960s to cover older people who were ever more frail, dependent and lacking mental capacity (Means and Smith, 1998a). This continued to be the case in the 1970s and 1980s, with particular concern being expressed by local authorities about the cost and staffing implications, as well as increasing frustration with the growing reluctance of the health service to enter into a dialogue about how best to respond to these challenges (see also Chapter Five).

The London Borough provides numerous examples of these worries during the early 1970s. In September 1971, a report on "staffing needs (care and attention) in homes for the elderly"[17] expressed concern about inadequate staffing levels given the range and prevalence of frailty and disability of residents as assessed by each matron, and went on to suggest that this was having a very deleterious impact on care provision:

> At present (the staff) are aware that they cannot give the standard of
> care which they wish to and the burden of this knowledge is added to
> the strain of the work. One matron admits that this strain sometimes
> results in lack of tolerance and undue briskness; another is concerned
> that some infirm residents are being put to bed earlier than is desirable;
> others speak of the inability to feel pride in the standards achieved[18]. .

The report goes on to discuss the daily routine of residents, but this is
done in a manner detached from the actual experiences and needs of the
residents. The focus is on how to improve the efficient use of staff time,
rather than on the quality of care available to those for whom a service is
being provided.

In December 1975, the Social Services Committee received a major
report on "dependency levels of residents in council homes for elderly
people"[19], a piece of research commissioned because of the need "to
document what was felt ... to be a changing role of the old people's
homes, within the overall context of health, social services and special
housing provision for elderly people"[20]. This looked at 483 residents in
10 local authority residential homes and found that two in five were over
85, one in five needed help in moving between rooms, one in nine were
doubly incontinent, significant numbers were either somewhat or severely
confused and considerable staff time was being consumed "in overseeing
the taking of drugs and providing some basic nursing care for the
residents"[21].

The main conclusion of the report was that "social services are carrying
a heavy load in giving residential care to the elderly and that assistance
from the health authority is required in the form of community nursing
services, provision of training facilities, provision of more full time nursing
care, and so on"[22]. Such help was not forthcoming.

Very similar debates and concerns can be traced in County Council
(B)[23]. In September 1972, the Social Services Committee was told about
the need to increase staffing levels because of increased levels of "infirmity,
disability and disturbance observed in residents"[24]. A survey organised
by the Deputy County Medical Officer of the "physical and mental frailty
of residents of old people's homes" confirmed this observation, with 67.6%
of residents having some physical impairment, 79.2% some form of
dementia or mental health problem and 22.3% requiring daily or weekly
nursing care[25]. The findings were felt to raise some major issues about the
responsibilities of the health service as opposed to social services:

If a higher proportion of sick, mentally frail and terminal cases need care in our homes, both staffing ratios and availability of staff with nursing qualifications may need to be considered, as well as the type of accommodation provided. If such change is thought to affect the character of our homes so as to change their function, is it appropriate that the local authority should continue to carry responsibility or should there be some re-shuffling between the local authority and hospitals[26].

As with the London Borough, the fairness of the health and social care boundary was being queried. Was the health service pushing too many older people with health care problems into local authority residential care?

A similar argument can be found in the committee reports of County Council (C). In March 1977, the Director of Social Services was offering enthusiastic support for plans to be developed by Area Health Authorities (AHAs) as part of new NHS planning systems[27] in the belief that this was likely to force AHAs to recognise the deficiencies of NHS provision for older people. These deficiencies had been specified in a report resulting from a joint visit by the Health Advisory Service and the Social Work Service of the Department of Health and Social Security. This had noted the strain placed on local authority residential care by the "shortage of continuing care psychogeriatric beds in the Health Service"[28]. However, social services were also concerned about the need to review staff ratios in residential homes because "the level of infirmity ... which they are expected to cope with steadily increases"[29].

Finally, the Metropolitan Authority was struggling with the same dilemmas. Although research carried out in 1975 had suggested a significant number of residents were capable of living in the community, if domiciliary support was available[30], the emphasis in the following two years remained the growing health problems of those in residential care:

... with the quite significant changes in the condition of elderly persons when admitted to homes, it has become increasingly difficult for staff. For much of the time in many of the homes, all staff can do is look after the physical needs of residents, ignoring their social and emotional needs. This leads to a reduction in the level of job satisfaction[31].

The situation was seen as being exacerbated by the challenge of working with those with dementia:

As the number of very elderly people increase so the number of confused elderly is increasing. At the moment, the authority has three homes for ambulant but confused, but difficulties are arising in the placement of confused residents either from their own homes or from hospital[32].

Recommendations included the establishment of a high dependency home, improved staff ratios and some regrading/reclassification of posts to reflect increased responsibilities and work pressures.

The overall impression given by the material explored in this section is that a problem is being recognised, but that the starting point is often not the quality of life of the older resident. Rather, the focus is either on conflict with the health service or on staffing levels and work schedules. Typical of the latter is how members of the Social Services Committee from County Council (C) were given profiles of staff deployment in one of their homes:

> *Old People's Home* (59 residents) visited at 2.30pm. The Deputy on duty had been discussing individual residents with visiting general practitioner from 1.45 to 2.30pm.

> An Assistant Head was attending a resident who appeared to have fallen.

> A Care Assistant was preparing tables for tea and attending to the needs of a resident who had been an outpatient at hospital and was having a late lunch.

> At the time of the visit, one resident was confined to bed, two care staff were about to come on duty and would need briefing, and one care staff was soon to go off duty. With an overall care staff of 1 to 9.65 there was, in fact, 1 to 19 and all of the three actually on duty were engaged with individuals[33].

Even more explicit was a report on work schedules from the London Borough, which admitted that "to wake everyone at 6.30am is not ideal but to leave it later means that the help of the night staff is lost during one of the day's heaviest periods of work"[34].

Conflict with the health service over this issue continued to rumble on and early developments in joint finance programmes were often used to tackle the problem. One frequent outcome was the development of a newly built residential home, designed and staffed to provide a service for older people with dementia or others with high dependency needs (see

Chapter Five). However, such capital investments did nothing to clarify the changing role of the rest of the local authority residential care homes.

Overall, the frailty and declining health of many older residents was thus often presented in a negative light, even if this was usually implied rather than overt. They were a source of conflict with the health service and they created staffing problems in residential homes. They were even a source of tension between residents:

> ... residents who are reasonably sound in mind and body find it difficult to accept the relatively poor social standards of frail disturbed old people and to share with them dining tables and chairs[35].

The general conclusion has to be that this was a period of more talk than action. The training of residential staff was not transformed and very little capital investment was going into existing residential homes as part of refurbishment programmes. What is not in doubt was that pressures on local authority residential care were increasing. The 1981 White Paper, *Growing older* (DHSS, 1981c), pointed out that older people used to enter such care in their sixties, but that the average age was now approaching 82 years with "an increasing number of residents (who) are mentally infirm or have physical disabilities" (p 45). The previous consultation document, *A happier old age* (DHSS, 1978a) noted how "... local authorities have ... been asked to find room within a reduced capital programme for more residential homes to meet increasing local needs" (p 29). But what about the impact of the spectacular growth of independent sector residential and nursing home care from 1983 onwards? How would this affect local authority residential care?

Responding to the challenge of the independent sector

Amendments were made to supplementary benefit regulations in the early 1980s in order to even out the opportunities for the low-income residents of private and voluntary residential and nursing homes to claim their fees from the social security system. Such individuals were assessed only in terms of financial entitlement, and no check was introduced on their need for such care (Means and Smith, 1998b, Chapter Three). Provision in the independent sector (and especially private homes) mushroomed from 49,900 places in 1982 to 161,200 places in 1991 (Laing and Buisson, 1992, p 156), with the vast bulk of homes being for older people.

The public expenditure consequences of this development were considerable. In 1979, 11,000 claimants were claiming only £10 million from the social security system. By the time of the implementation of the main community care reforms, the number of claimants had risen to 281,200 and they were receiving £2.6 billion (Laing and Buisson, 1994; Player and Pollock, 2001;Tinker, 1997). This is why so many commentators have argued that the community care reforms brought in by the 1990 Act were really about "the need to stop the haemorrhage in the social security budget" (Lewis and Glennerster, 1996, p 8). This was of course to be achieved by asking local authorities to assess people for such care in terms of both need and entitlement, and to do this within finite budgets (see Chapter One).

How did all of this affect our four case studies? In terms of crude provision in the private sector, the answer is in strikingly different ways. Table 4.1 profiles residential provision in 1985 and 1990, and illustrates not only the speed of growth of this sector but also how County Council (B) had one of the largest private sectors in the country, while the London Borough had one of the smallest. These differences become even more marked when private sector nursing home places are added, since they totalled over 4,000 places in County Council (B) in 1990 and well under 100 for the London Borough. Indeed, the number of places in private

Table 4.1: Number of places in residential homes for older people (31 March 1985 and 31 March 1990)

Local authority	Local authority homes	Voluntary homes	Private homes	Total
31 March 1985				
London Borough	324	91	9	424
County Council (B)	2,275	769	6,422	9,466
County Council (C)	1,137	188	327	1,652
Metropolitan Authority	629	35	433	1,097
31 March 1990				
London Borough	393	124	16	533
County Council (B)	1,976	976	10,234	13,186
County Council (C)	1,217	309	813	2,339
Metropolitan Authority	578	36	665	1,279

Sources: DHSS (1985 and 1990) *Personal social services local authority statistics: Residential accommodation for elderly and younger handicapped people – all residents in local authority and private homes*. Years ending 31 March 1985 (RA/85/2) Tables 2, 4 and 5, and year ending 31 March 1990 (RA/90/2) Table 2.

Table 4.2: Number of places in voluntary and private sector nursing homes in 1987 and 1990

1987

Health authority area	Voluntary sector homes		Private sector homes	
	Number of health authority registered places in single and jointly registered homes	Number of local authority registered places in jointly registered homes	Number of health authority registered places in single and jointly registered homes	Number of local authority registered places in jointly registered homes
London Borough	39	73	180	82
County Council (B)	147	7	2,485	56
County Council (C)	102	111	467	47
Metropolitan Authority	209	0	377	0

1990

Health authority area	Voluntary sector homes		Private sector homes	
	Number of health authority registered places in single and jointly registered homes	Number of local authority registered places in jointly registered homes	Number of health authority registered places in single and jointly registered homes	Number of local authority registered places in jointly registered homes
London Borough	89	73	85	0
County Council (B)	187	38	4,020	221
County Council (C)	132	110	859	113
Metropolitan Authority	45	0	730	15

Sources: *Laing's review of private healthcare and directory of independent hospitals, nursing and residential homes and related services,* London: Laing & Buisson Publications Ltd, 1987 and 1990

sector nursing homes in the London Borough went down from 180 in 1987 to under 100 in 1990 (see Table 4.2).

The likely reasons for this are not hard to decipher. County Council (B) had a large population of older people, it was popular as a place to retire to and its large number of coastal resorts contained numerous failing hotels, which were suitable for conversion to residential or nursing homes. The London Borough on the other hand was an area with relatively few large buildings, where both property and land prices were very high. County Council (C) and the Metropolitan Authority fell very much between these two extremes in terms of both demography and the availability of suitable property.

One consequence of these developments was a further review of the role of local authority residential homes. However, this was not a simple result of the growth of alternative provision in receipt of a higher public subsidy than local authority residential care. It also arose from concern about the quality of local authority provision when measured against the requirements for the independent sector under the 1984 Registered Homes Act and the associated good practice guidance, *Home life* (Avebury, 1984).

It would be wrong to argue that *Home life* was the only factor in generating a quality debate in terms of local authority residential care. The influential research by Willcocks et al (1987), *Private lives in public places*, had argued that residents lacked adequate privacy and this could be provided by developing residential flatlets (see also, Willcocks et al, 1982). This had a significant impact on Department of Health thinking (Judge and Sinclair, 1986). In 1985, Norman Fowler as Secretary of State for Health and Social Services commissioned an independent review of residential care across all sectors and all client groups. The emphasis of the resultant Wagner Report (1988) was on residential care as "a positive choice" for some and one where the rights of residents required much more emphasis than in the past. However, it will be seen below that it was *Home life* (1984), and the use of it by government to influence the local authority sector, which had the deepest impact on the four case studies.

The 1984 Registered Homes Act covered independent sector residential care homes in Part One of the Act (to be registered with the local authority) and independent nursing homes in Part Two (to be registered with the health authority). With regard to the former, registration and inspection procedures were laid out in detailed regulations sent to all local authorities and were combined with the government supported good practice code, *Home life* (Avebury, 1984). The code contained separate sections on the principles of care, social care, physical features, the needs of individual client groups, staff and the role of the registration authority.

Although the Act, the regulations and *Home life* applied only to private and voluntary homes, an early response from proprietors was that the same yardsticks of fitness and good practice should apply to local authority residential homes (Peace et al, 1997). Were local authority residents afforded such basic rights as fulfilment, the preservation of self-respect and the right to self-determination rather than regimentation? Did admission procedures include home brochures, introductory visits and trial stays? Were there clear written statements of terms and conditions, including complaints procedures? Did residents in local authority homes have their own room (unless requested otherwise) in order to foster privacy and personal autonomy? Were fire regulations adequate? Did local authority residents have adequate access to toilets and bathrooms? Did their homes have adequate central heating? Were there adequate facilities and adaptations for disabled older residents? Were staffing arrangements adequate? Did these premises feel like a home or an institution? After all, such questions were to be asked of the independent sector on a regular basis.

A number of factors ensured that local authorities could not ignore such challenges. First, residential and nursing home proprietors were often well organised locally with strong links to local politicians (especially those sympathetic to the private sector as a social care provider) and the local press. Second, the White Paper, *Caring for people* (DoH, 1989a) proposed that social services authorities should set up independent inspection and registration units that were at arms length from local authority providers. Such units would inspect both local authority and independent sector homes, all to the same standards.

Finally, the Social Services Inspectorate of the Department of Health was emphasising the need to push public sector residential care towards *Home life* standards prior to it becoming subject to the same regulatory standards. The Social Services Inspectorate produced *Towards a climate of confidence* (Social Services Inspectorate, 1989), which contained 11 key recommendations to help local authorities deliver (and monitor) high quality care in local authority residential homes. They included:

- officers in charge and their immediate line managers should receive management training;
- greater autonomy at the level of the home should be created by delegating budgets, with appropriate controls and regular information feedback;

- clear brochures for homes, setting out what the home can offer, associated with a charter of rights for residents;
- a statement of how to make a complaint, where and to whom;
- care plans, clearly recorded and agreed with residents or their supporters, routinely received;
- clear standards by which to evaluate performance;
- a system of inspection of homes carried out independently of line management systems.

Such guidance was telling local authorities that they were now in a market for residential care customers, and that this needed to be reflected in all aspects of local authority residential provision.

One might expect the London Borough to be little affected by the *Home life* debate, given the lack of a private sector. This was not the case. As early as July 1988, the Social Services Committee agreed the complete refurbishment of one home as part of its move towards *Home life* standards of care and support. Several works were approved and the Committee also agreed to reduce the number of residents from 39 to 24[36].

This local authority had closed two homes in 1989/90 as part of general cost cutting exercises[37]. However, it was committed to tackle the *Home life* agenda for the rest of its stock, partly because of some major difficulties that had arisen in one particular home. In October 1990, the Social Services Committee considered a paper on standards and management in residential homes for older people[38]. This went through the 11 key recommendations of the *Towards a climate of confidence* report (Social Services Inspectorate, 1989), and profiled how the authority was responding to each of them. For example, under the recommendation on brochures and the charter of rights, it was confirmed that information packs were available from January 1991, while "a Charter of Rights for residents was agreed by Social Services Committee in April 1990"[39]. On the evaluation of standards, it was stressed that "much effort during the past five years has been put into establishing the principles of the *Home life* code of practice as the basic standards of the council's residential homes"[40]. A number of in-house training events had been run for residential staff on *Home life* principles and their practical application.

The extent of this effort demonstrates that the London Borough expected to remain the dominant provider of residential care. Not only was there a real shortage of independent sector provision (only one home within the borough), but there was a political commitment from the ruling Labour group to the importance of local authority provision, rather than to contracting out homes to a third party. This meant that members were more willing than in the other three case study areas to support upgrading for all the remaining local authority homes. Substantial capital monies were set aside from the late 1980s onwards[41]. This major refurbishment of homes for older people meant "an awful lot of capital was spent which 'unitised' every single residential establishment" (interview with Director of Social Services [A], 1986-1994) (that is, all multiply occupied rooms were finally removed).

County Council (B) faced a major challenge about what to do with its in-house provision given that (i) it was in desperate need of refurbishment and (ii) there was a massive independent sector available for older people to choose from. Concern about the quality of the local authority provision can be traced back at least to the early 1980s when the Director of Social Services was asking his committee to accept "the principle that there should be no more than three persons to a bedroom in its own old people's homes"[42]. He also reflected that "some ... homes are made up ... of shared or multi occupancy rooms, and one must begin to question the extent to which these homes can meet the needs of very frail and handicapped residents"[43]. This was seen as especially problematic, since the growth of private homes had greatly reduced waiting lists for local authority homes and suggested their future role might be a specialist one focused on those deemed most dependent[44]. The existing stock was not well suited to this new role.

The situation was reassessed in June 1986, as a result of a report from a review team on "residential homes for the elderly and hostels for the mentally handicapped"[45]. Drawing on a model and philosophy of good care practice associated with *Home life*, it was claimed that "the quality of care in the best County Council establishments matched that which may be found in the very best of the private sector"[46]. The way forward was to integrate such provision within locality plans as part of a continuum of care. The objective was to enable them to "become 'resource centres' closely identified with the communities they serve whence families and neighbours may seek and obtain advice, and offering the use of facilities to other establishments and the community as a whole"[47]. It was recognised that this would require an upgrading of many of the homes, combined with extensive staff training.

However, pressure for more radical change continued to grow. The option of transfer of all or some of the Council's residential homes was considered[48] and occupancy levels continued to fall ("partly because of the uncertainty surrounding the future of the homes"[49]). The mass transfer of homes was rejected on the grounds of uncertainty about future funding arrangements as a result of the Griffiths Report (1988). Instead, the emphasis on locality/district planning remained, but this time with a much sharper edge. The planning task at district level was to identify "the least viable homes in care, financial and property terms"[50] with a view to their subsequent closure.

In April 1989, the Conservatives gained control of the local authority and decided the process of home closure needed to be speeded up for the following reasons:

> We did have a ball park figure of around £15 to £20 million to bring them up to scratch. Even to provide the basic things like fire door closures and to reduce the number of multiple rooms down. When I went round the homes it was quite common to see four or five beds in a room. Mostly double sharing rooms, very few singles. No en suite facilities whatsoever. Lino floors. Typical institutionalised types of homes which I don't think was satisfactory. (interview with Chair of the Social Services Committee [B], 1989-93)

It was decided to push forward a major programme of home closures with the intention of reducing the overall number of local authority homes from 55 homes in late 1988 to 39 by April 1993[51]. Money saved from the closures was to be reinvested in the remaining homes to bring them up to registration standard, and hence able to offer the following services: (a) long-term care of people with high levels of dependency, that is, mentally ill older people, the most frail and handicapped older people, and those with challenging patterns of behaviour; and (b) respite care and rehabilitation/assessment purposes[52]. Money saved from the closures was thus used to improve local authority services with an emphasis on what the Director of Social Services from January 1990 onwards called "reablement services" (interview with Director of Social Services [B], 1990-99).

However, such a large programme of closures proved enormously controversial, especially in 1990 when nine homes were put forward as no longer viable. These closures were bitterly opposed by the other political parties and by the trades unions, with a heavy emphasis from opponents that the Council was closing down the homes of very vulnerable people. The then Director of Social Services remembers decision day at the Council generating "one of the biggest demonstrations of all time in this County Council" (interview with Director of Social Services [B], 1990-99), as well as 60,000 letters of protest. Even after the closure decision was made, opponents took the decision all the way to judicial review. (The Council won its case on the grounds that residents had been properly consulted within a planned programme of closure, although another county lost its case because of the failure to do this.)

County Council (C) had significant in-house provision of residential care (27 homes in 1990), but also a sizeable independent sector. By 1990, it was carrying out an extensive review of the local authority provision for a number of interlocking reasons[53]:

- to upgrade local authority homes for older people in line with *Home life* standards;
- to refocus such homes as catering "for the most physically and mentally frail elderly people"[54];
- to ensure overall residential provision reflected the demographic spread of older people in the County;
- to ensure additional resources were released for the continuing support of older people in their own homes.

In order to achieve these objectives, a working party undertook "a detailed evaluation of the work required and the cost and feasibility of bringing each of the council's homes up to acceptable standards for frail elderly people"[55]. The working party concluded that five homes should be closed (all were old converted houses with modern brick extensions, inadequate lifts and numerous shared rooms). The resultant capital receipts would contribute to the cost of (i) upgrading the remaining 23 homes; and (ii) the building of an extra care sheltered housing scheme to be run by a housing association.

Such ambitious plans for modernisation proved difficult to implement in the context of public expenditure restrictions in general and controls on capital projects in particular. A report in March 1992 was talking in terms of a £10.8 million capital investment for a refurbishment programme of 12 homes (two homes to be upgraded each year) in a context where the then capital programme was already showing a shortfall of £8 million in the period to 1995-96[56]. By September 1993, only six local authority homes were meeting registration standards and the local authority continued to struggle to find the capital investment to drive forward its expensive refurbishment programme[57].

The Director of Social Services for this period referred to the problem of resolving the local authority residential homes issue as "my biggest failure" (interview with Director of Social Services [C], 1988-1995). He recalled how bad conditions were in those homes, which had been converted from large country houses:

They took me to this stable block and downstairs there was nothing, so we had to go up these stairs and upstairs … there were five, what I would call cells in it…. I went into one and there was this old (man) there and he was blind. And he had the tinniest … radio you've ever seen with a bit of wire stuck to the wall, a bed with an iron frame and a wardrobe that looked like it'd come off the scrap heap. (interview with Director of Social Services [C], 1988–95)

The 'stables' were being used to accommodate older men with a history of homelessness. However, the Director felt "it was an absolute disgrace" and decided that it must be closed as soon as possible.

Other homes, and especially those that had been purpose-built, were deemed worth upgrading. However, because of the lack of available capital monies, he had tried to get the agreement of the Council to transfer such homes to an independent organisation. This was attempted five years running with "rows in council chambers" and "TV cameras outside County Hall" (interview with Director of Social Services [C], 1988–95). Each time this option was rejected, but in the end "the worst homes did get closed eventually, one at a time, through individual bloodbaths" (interview with Director of Social Services [C], 1988–95). Opposition to both closure and transfer came from the Labour group on the Council and the trades unions.

The Metropolitan Authority considered the issue of multi-bedded accommodation in its residential homes for older people as early as 1982. A review looked at the older purpose-built accommodation and the adapted properties where rooms were shared by up to six residents. However, the cost of adaptation, combined with the resultant loss of beds, led to a recommendation "that as a result of the feasibility study, no further action be taken to sub-divide existing bedrooms in elderly persons' homes at the present time"[58].

Such a position was not sustainable. During the mid-1980s, the Social Services Committee received a number of reports relating to older people. These pointed out the need for local authority provision to reflect *Home life* standards and for the Council to be clear on the role of its own provision in the light of the growth of the private sector (independent sector residential home places had risen from 23 homes with 263 places in December 1981 to 40 homes with 575 places in Autumn 1986[59]). As a result, there was "much debate about how much residential care should be provided by the council"[60] and specific decisions made about the closure of those homes with the poorest physical standards (one of these had eight residents to a room), the upgrading of others (especially to reduce multi-occupancy), redesignation of some homes as "high dependence"[61] only, and an exploration of the potential of local authority homes as locality resource centres. A District Officer for social services for this period remembers provision in the mid-1980s needed radical overhaul, since "shared rooms were the norm", "very little money was spent on furniture" and there was "a rather patronising attitude" to residents (interview with Senior Social Services Manager [D], 1985-93).

As with other case studies, the end result of all this debate and effort was still that "many of the existing council owned residential homes do not come up to the registration standards required ... but the capital programme could not enable us to upgrade all the homes until well into the next century"[62]. The option of transferring the bulk of the homes to an independent company was initially rejected. The viability of this venture was not clear and in any case such a transfer would reduce the ability of the local authority to shift resources from residential care to the support of people in their own homes. Instead, the following course of action was proposed:

> ... the only viable way forward is to change the role of some elderly persons' homes to that of sheltered housing units, with the Division continuing to care for the tenants in such units; to offer for sale a small number of units not suitable for such redevelopment, to upgrade the remaining homes to registration standards ... and to redefine the role of the remaining homes concentrating on respite and rehabilitation care. At the same time, and using all the finances released by this course of action, home care services must be extended and developed[63].

In short, the proposal was that local authority residential care for older people should be dramatically downsized, a suggestion that worried many councillors and provoked the hostility of the trades unions because of concern "about the future employment of their members"[64].

Such opposition and doubt seemed to have led to a policy rethink, although one still committed to radical change. In the end, the Council did decide to remain a direct provider through the retention of six homes[65], which reflected the geographical spread of the borough, and to close one additional home. However, the remaining nine homes were to be transferred to two independent organisations[66], although this again met with fierce opposition from the trades unions (interview with Senior Social Services Manager [D], 1985-93).

Conclusion

Local authority residential care has been strongly criticised for a long time. This chapter helps to explain why such a heavy emphasis on building new residential homes existed in the early 1970s and has examined how four social services authorities responded to the increasing age, ill health and infirmity of residents. However, the late 1970s and early 1980s was also a period of neglect for such homes in terms of physical standards and often in terms of the quality of care. These deficiencies were exposed by the rapid development of independent sector residential and nursing home care in the 1980s and the associated passing of the 1984 Registered Homes Act and publication of *Home life* (Avebury, 1984). The four social services authorities did their best to respond to this situation. All made real attempts to improve the quality of care, but three decided that the only way forward was the transfer or closure of many of their homes and all three found themselves in what one Director of Social Services called "EPH wars" (interview with Director of Social Services [C], 1988-95). Overall, the harsh conclusion is that perhaps most local authorities did "too little, too late" to ensure most of their own homes would have a long-term future in the mixed economy of residential care.

Notes

[1] Social Services Committee (A), 23 October 1972 (Progress on Capital Works).

[2] Social Services Committee (B), 8 December 1971 (Estimates of Capital Expenditure 1971/72 to 1974/75).

[3] Social Services Committee (C), 28 May 1975 (Budget Plans, Manpower Planning and the Public Expenditure White Paper).

[4] Social Services Committee (D), 16 February 1976 (Social Services Capital Building Programme, 1976/77).

[5] Social Services Committee (A), 8 December 1975 (Occupancy of Home for the Elderly: Proposed Reduction in Places Available).

[6] Social Services Committee (C) 12 December 1971 (Allocation of Places in Old People's Homes).

[7] Social Services Committee (B), 9 December 1982 (Bedroom Accommodation in Old People's Homes).

[8] Social Services Committee (D), 25 January 1977 (Policy Options, 1977-78).

[9] Social Services Committee (B), 2 September 1975 (Priorities for the Social Services Department).

[10] Social Services Committee (D), 7 June 1988 (Capital Programme).

[11] Social Services Committee (B), 17 September 1981 (1981/82 Capital Programme).

[12] Social Services Committee (A), 28 July 1975 (Future Level of Expenditure Plans).

[13] Social Services Committee (B), 17 September 1981 (1981/82 Capital Programme).

[14] Social Services Committee (C), 10 December 1976 (Capital Programme 1976/ 77 to 1980/81).

[15] Social Services Committee (D), 16 February 1976 (Capital Building Programme, 1976/77).

[16] Social Services Committee (C), 10 March 1977 (Expenditure in Residential Establishments).

[17] Social Services Committee (A), 13 September 1971 (Interim Report on Staffing Needs [Care and Attention] in Homes for the Elderly).

[18] Ibid.

[19] Social Services Committee (A), 8 December 1975 (Dependency Levels of Residents in Council Homes for the Elderly).

[20] Ibid.

[21] Ibid.

[22] Ibid.

[23] Social Services Committee (B), 13 September 1972 (Staffing).

[24] Ibid.

[25] Social Services Committee (B), 6 December 1972 (Medical Survey in Homes for the Elderly).

[26] Ibid.

[27] Social Services Committee (C), 18 March 1977 (Area Health Authority – Creation of First Health Area Plan).

[28] Social Services Committee (C), 11 September 1981 (Commentary by the

Director of Social Services on a Report of a Visit by the Health Advisory Service and Social Work Service of DHSS).

[29] Social Services Committee (C), 18 March 1977 (Deployment of Caring Staff in Residential Establishments).

[30] Social Services Committee (D), March 1976 (The Elderly: A Policy Report).

[31] Social Services Committee (D), 6 June 1978 (Staffing in Residential Establishments).

[32] Ibid.

[33] Social Services Committee (C), 18 March 1977 (Deployment of Caring Staff in Residential Establishments).

[34] Social Services Committee (A), 3 January 1974 (Residential Care Staff in Old People's Homes).

[35] Social Services Committee (B), 6 December 1972 (Medical Survey in Homes for the Elderly).

[36] Social Services Committee (A), 11 July 1988 (Multi Year Capital Programme, 1987/88 to 1989/90).

[37] Social Services Committee (A), 27 April 1990 (Key Strategic Issues for Social Services in 1990/91).

[38] Social Services Committee (A), 22 October 1990 (Standards and Management in Residential Homes for Elderly People).

[39] Ibid.

[40] Ibid.

[41] Social Services Committee (A), 31 January 1989 (Revised Estimated 1989-90).

[42] Social Services Committee (B), 9 December 1982 (Bedroom Accommodation in Old People's Homes).

[43] Ibid.

[44] Social Services Committee (B), 8 December 1983 (Residential Care for the Elderly – A Policy for the Future).

[45] Social Services Committee (B), 19 June 1986 (Departmental Review: Residential Homes for the Elderly and Hostels for the Mentally Handicapped).

[46] Ibid.

[47] Ibid.

[48] Social Services Committee (B), 7 April 1988 (Proposed Charitable Trust for Homes for the Elderly).

[49] Social Services Committee (B), 23 June 1988 (Revenue Budget, 1988/89).

[50] Social Services Committee (B), 23 June 1988 (The Future of Homes for the Elderly).

[51] Social Services Committee (B), 1 February 1990 (Report of the Homes for the Elderly Working Party).

[52] Ibid.

[53] Social Services Committee (C), 16 January 1990 (Care of the Elderly Strategy – Residential Provision).

[54] Ibid.

[55] Ibid.

[56] Social Services Committee (C), 3 March 1992 (Services for Elderly People – Home Refurbishment Standard).

[57] Social Services Committee (C), 28 September 1993 (Homes for Elderly People Development Programme).

[58] Social Services Committee (D), 23 March 1982 (Multi-bedded Accommodation in Elderly Persons' Homes).

[59] Social Services Committee (D), 25 November 1986 (Residential and Day Care for Elderly People).

[60] Ibid.

[61] Ibid.

[62] Social Services Committee (D), 29 May 1990 (Care of Elderly People).

[63] Ibid.

[64] Ibid.

[65] Social Services Committee (D), 28 May 1991 (Services for Elderly People).

[66] Social Services Committee (D), 14 January 1992 (Services for Elderly People: Transfer of Elderly Persons Homes).

FIVE

The shifting boundaries between health and social care

Introduction

Any study of the development of welfare services for older people in the 1971-93 period must consider the interface between social services and health, a point already made clear in the previous chapter in terms of how health services were often the driving force behind changes in local authority residential care. This period was one of sustained exhortation from central government on the need to work together across the two agencies, but also one of enormous organisational change for health.

This chapter begins by offering a short review of some of these key policy and organisational changes and goes on to explore how health-social services relationships worked themselves out in the four case study authorities. Like other themes in this book, many of the same issues were to be found in all the localities. More specifically, there was constant tension over 'what is health care?' and 'what is social care?', with the fear on the part of social services that health was pushing more and more responsibilities for older people their way without any significant transfer of resources.

The policy and organisational context

Three years after the creation in 1971 of social services departments in English local authorities, there was a major reorganisation of both the local government system and the NHS. For both services, it was argued that major changes were required to improve efficiency and effectiveness and for the NHS in particular, reorganisation would achieve these objectives through greater integration. Fourteen Regional Health Authorities were established within which there were 90 Area Health Authorities. Under the Area Health Authorities, there were 205 District Management Teams. Domiciliary health care services, such as home nursing and health visiting, previously the responsibility of local authorities, were transferred to the NHS. In mirror image, medical/hospital social work was shifted from the NHS to local authority social services departments. At the same time the Executive Councils, which had administered the services provided by general practitioners, dentists, opticians and pharmacists, were replaced by 90 Family Practitioner Committees. Community Health Councils were created at District Management Team level to represent the views of interest groups and the users of health services (see Brown, 1979).

Between 1974 and 1993, the overall responsibility for the range of domiciliary and day health care services in support of vulnerable older people remained as determined in 1974. However, the management and structure of the NHS during this period underwent further transformations, requiring in turn reconsideration by local authorities of the best way to work with health care colleagues.

The 1974 NHS reforms were soon seen not to be producing the desired results of increased efficiency and effectiveness and the multi-tiered system was constantly criticised. One of the recommendations in the report of the Royal Commission on the NHS (1979) was that one of the levels of management under the Regional Health Authorities should disappear. Following a consultation paper, *Patients first* (DHSS and the Welsh Office, 1979), the government introduced the 1980 Health Service Act, under which the 90 Area Health Authorities and the 200 plus District Management Teams were replaced by 192 District Health Authorities, even though the Area Health Authorities had in the main coterminous boundaries with the reorganised local authorities, which were responsible for social services. Soon after this, in February 1983, the Griffiths Management Inquiry Team began its work and rapidly completed a final report in October of the same year. The report took the form of a letter to the Secretary of State and recommended the replacement of consensus management by a system of general management (Griffiths, 1983). This was accepted by the government, which required the District Health Authorities to appoint general managers at all levels by the end of 1985.

These management changes had their main impact on hospitals. Proposals for changes in primary health care were published in the mid-1980s (DHSS, 1987), underpinned by ideas of preventive medicine and health promotion. Large general practices could choose to become fundholders. The new arrangements were built into the 1990 NHS and Community Care Act and came into force in April 1991. The former Family Practitioner Committees were turned into Family Health Services Authorities and made accountable to Regional Health Authorities.

This same legislation brought further changes to the organisation of hospital and community health services following a funding crisis and another review of the NHS leading to a White Paper, *Working for patients* (DoH, 1989b). The idea of the purchaser/provider split, promoted by American health economist, Alain Enthoven (1985), was introduced in April 1991. The implementation of this change goes beyond 1993, but suffice it to say that the government recognised that further structural reform was needed to make sense of the introduction of the internal market and following the 1995 Health Authorities Act, 100 Health Authorities and over 400 NHS Hospital and Community Health Trusts were created in April 1996. The 100 Health Authorities brought together the former Family Health Services Authorities and the District Health Authorities.

Implementation of the community care reforms of the 1990 Act was put off until April 1993 and local authority social services departments found themselves planning radical change in terms of their regulatory and service delivery responsibilities at the same time as a further upheaval in one of its key partners, the NHS. Over the 1971 to 1993 period, the emphasis shifted from structural to processual changes to the NHS. But what about changes in the thrust of policy over these 22 years? And what kinds of health policy initiatives over the 1971 to 1993 period had particular consequences for frail older people? The cost of the NHS had been a matter for official concern since its inception, and the recession and the squeeze on public expenditure in the mid-1970s added to the pressures. Criteria for the allocation of scarce resources in different regions of England included demographic factors such as the proportion of older people, and emphasis was placed on prevention in the planning of services and resources (DHSS, 1976a). This theme was reflected in the 1979 report of the Royal Commission on the National Health Service, set up in 1976 to consider the best use and management of the financial and labour resources of the NHS. In 1976, the government also issued a consultation document, *Priorities for health and personal social services in England* (DHSS, 1976b), and introduced joint finance arrangements.

The 1973 NHS Reorganisation Act had established machinery for joint planning between health and local authorities through member-based Joint Consultative Committees. One of the main purposes of this initiative was to plan for the rundown of long stay hospitals and the encouragement of community-based services for a range of people, including frail older people. White Papers on better services for people with mental health problems and/or learning difficulties were published in 1971 and 1975, whereas discussion rather than policy documents was the order of the day for older people (DHSS, 1976c, 1976d, 1978a).

The joint planning arrangements failed to make good progress, so joint finance was introduced as an incentive. The arrangement was that, for a limited period, social services departments could receive health authority funds to underpin community-based services for people leaving long stay hospitals or to support people so that they would not seek hospital based support. This mechanism formed part of the way forward in addressing health and social services priorities published in 1977 (DHSS, 1977) and in a discussion document on collaboration in community care produced the following year (DHSS, 1978b).

The Royal Commission report, published in 1979, came soon after the election of a Conservative government with Mrs Thatcher as Prime Minister. It recognised the importance of providing, if possible, care in the community for vulnerable older people and again highlighted the problem of shifting resources to achieve this goal. The recommendations of the Royal Commission were accepted in part by the new administration and early in 1981 it issued guidance for health and personal social services (DHSS, 1981a) and a White Paper on a policy for older people, *Growing older* (DHSS, 1981c). The former included frail older people among its priorities with the by now familiar emphasis on care for people in their own homes and on rehabilitation of those in hospital, as well as recognising that the need for long-term care in an institutional setting would not completely disappear. This message was echoed in the White Paper, *Growing older*.

Later in 1981 a consultative document was published on moving resources for care beyond the arrangements embedded in joint finance (DHSS, 1981b). This focused in particular on the transfer of people from long stay hospitals and put forward a wide range of options, including the handover of buildings, the movement of funds between government departments, lump sum payments, allowing local authority housing departments or housing associations to receive joint financing and extending the period of eligibility for joint financing from 7 to 13 years. Some of the proposals were seen as quite radical, but were in the end not adopted. A March 1983 government circular announced a modest increase in funds, longer periods of funding and an extension of joint finance to cover education and housing projects. A pilot programme on care in the community, which took the form of demonstration projects, was promoted with special DHSS funds, and voluntary sector representatives were encouraged to join health and local authority members on Joint Consultative Committees (DHSS, 1983). Whilst the 1981 consultative document concentrated on ways of moving people out of long stay hospitals, reports were also published in the same year on the impact on acute hospital provision of lack of investment in geriatric departments and on the fact that most of the increase in demand for acute beds was coming from the older population (DHSS, 1981d, 1981e).

By the mid-1980s the main policy focus was on the health and social care interface (Audit Commission, 1986; DHSS, 1985; House of Commons Social Services Committee, 1985) and on primary health care (DHSS, 1986a, 1986b, 1987; House of Commons Social Services Committee, 1987). Meanwhile, the NHS was experiencing further funding crises that led to a further review of the service and the eventual introduction of the purchaser/provider split embedded in the 1990 NHS and Community Care Act.

Defining in need of care and attention, 1948-71

This short review of policy developments in the health service from 1971 to 1993 illustrates the growing concern of government about the health and social care interface. Chapter Four indicated the extent to which our case studies felt that they were being 'dumped upon' by health in terms of expectations about the kind of residents who should be in local authority residential care.

At the heart of many of these disputes and tensions lies ambiguity about what is meant by the term being 'in need of care and attention' under the 1948 National Assistance Act. When introducing the Bill to the House of Commons, Bevan (Minister of Health) said that the new residential homes were for "the type of old person who are still able to look after themselves ... but who are unable to do the housework, the laundry, cook meals and things of that sort" (*Hansard*, House of Commons, vol 443, no 24, 24 November 1947, col 1609). Although neither the Act nor the accompanying circulars gave an unambiguous definition of 'care and attention', Godlove and Mann (1980) were quite clear that "the authors ... of this Act ... did not envisage this type of care as being adequate for people suffering from incontinence, serious loss of mobility, or abnormal senile dementia" (p 4).

By the mid-1950s, local authorities felt their residential homes contained numerous older people who should really be in hospital care (Parker, 1965), while Hospital Boards felt they had beds blocked by the refusal of these authorities to carry out their statutory duties under the 1948 National Assistance Act. Their main disputes focused on a group of older people who were "stranded in the no man's land between the Regional Hospital Board and the local welfare department – not ill enough for one, not well enough for the other" (Huws Jones, 1952, pp 19-22).

The late 1950s and the 1960s saw numerous attempts to define the boundary between health and social care. As a result of the Boucher Report (1957) into health and welfare provision in later life, circulars were issued that set out the respective responsibilities of welfare and hospital authorities. Welfare authorities were informed that their duties included:

• care of the otherwise active resident in a welfare home during minor illness, which may well involve a short period in bed;
• care of the infirm (including the senile) who may need help in dressing, toilet, and so on, and may need to live on the ground floor because they cannot manage stairs, and may spend part of the day in bed (or longer periods in bad weather);
• care of those older persons in a welfare home who have to take to bed and are not expected to live more than a few weeks (or exceptionally months). Who would, if in their own homes, stay there because they cannot benefit from treatment or nursing care beyond help that can be given at home, and whose removal to hospital away from familiar surroundings and attendance would be felt to be inhumane (MoH, 1957a).

Hospital authorities, on the other hand, were expected to take responsibility for:

• care of the chronic bedfast who may need little or no medical treatment, but who do require prolonged nursing care over months or years;
• convalescent care of older sick people who have completed active treatment, but who are not yet ready for discharge to their own homes or to welfare homes;
• care of the senile confused or disturbed patients who are, owing to their mental condition, unfit to live a normal community life in a welfare home (MoH, 1957b).

Hospital authorities did not have responsibility to give "all medical or nursing care needed by an old person, however minor the illness or however short the stay in bed, nor to admit all those who need nursing care because they are entering on the last stage of their lives".

The 1957 circulars were updated in 1965 with an even stronger emphasis on the high level of dependency through frailty and ill health that a residential home should be able to cope with:

The elderly people whom (they) may need to admit or to retain in homes can broadly be described as those who are found, after careful assessment of their medical and social needs, to be unable to maintain themselves in their own homes, even with full support from outside, but who do not need continuous care by nursing staff. They include:

(i)   people so incapacitated that they need help with dressing, toilet and meals, but who are able to get about with a walking aid or with some help by wheelchair;

(ii)   people using appliances that they can manage themselves or without nursing assistance;

(iii) people with temporary or continuing confusion of mind but who do not need psychiatric nursing care.

They include also residents who fall ill, whether for short or long periods, whose needs are no greater than could be met in their own homes by relatives with the aid of the local health services. Where the illness is expected to be terminal, transfer to hospital should be avoided unless continuous medical or nursing care is necessary. Some incontinent residents (other than those with intractable incontinence and other disabilities) may also be manageable in a residential home. (MoH, 1965a, 1965b)

Local authority residential care had become 'home' to a very different group of people from that envisaged by the proponents of the 1948 Act. Attempts to clarify the boundary between health and social care had drawn a group into local authority care who were once seen as clearly having health care needs, which should be responded to free of charge through the health service (Means 2001; Means and Smith, 1998a). The rest of this chapter addresses the debate about the health and social care interface by examining developments in the four case study areas.

Reducing continuing care beds

It is hard to avoid the conclusion that one of the main drivers of community care policy for older people at a local level was the need for social services authorities to respond to major changes in health care provision. More specifically, in all four of our case studies (see Table 5.1) the NHS embarked upon significant reductions in long stay hospital beds for older people in line with national trends (Player and Pollock, 2001). This resulted in increasingly dependent residents in local authority residential care. The shift was also speeded up from the mid-1980s onwards by the growth in independent sector nursing home care (see Chapter Four). Another crucial factor was the lack of priority given by central government to long-term health care as opposed to acute care (DHSS, 1976b), combined with the national shortage of consultant geriatricians and psychogeriatricians (DHSS, 1981d).

The Social Services Committees of all four local authorities received a series of reports relating to concerns about inadequate 'continuing care' bed provision in the health service and the implications of this for social services. Thus, the London Borough had long argued for more rather than less 'continuing care' beds, and so in January 1977 they bemoaned how bed transfers from hospital closure "means the temporary abandonment of plans to increase the number of geriatric beds in the District"[1], while in January 1982, the Committee was concerned about the lack of consultation over the implications for social services of the closure of a large psychiatric hospital[2]. In a similar vein, the Director of Social Services for County Council (B) had called as early as June 1971 for "50 acute geriatric beds and a 30-bedded psychogeriatric assessment unit" together with 50 additional beds to be provided by small long stay units attached to existing general practitioner hospitals[3] in just one area of the County, and in September 1978 was complaining about a 513 geriatric bed deficit in another[4]. Perhaps the biggest difficulties related to the closure of the very large psychiatric hospitals, many of whose residents were older people. Although fully supportive of the policy, the local authority frequently complained about the failure to develop

Table 5.1: Hospital beds in case study authorities (1981 and 1991)

Case study	Beds in NHS hospital/ homes (psychiatric)		Beds in NHS hospital/ homes (other)	
	1981	1991	1981	1991
London Borough	76	–	2,229	473
County Council (B)	2,450	92	4,591	660
County Council (C)	1,639	326	2,992	531
Metropolitan Authority	88	145	1,818	176

Sources: Office of Population Censuses and Surveys (1982) Census 1981, County Reports, Part 1, London: HMSO, Table 9; Office of Population Censuses and Surveys (1992 and 1993) Census 1991, County Reports, Part 1, London: HMSO, Table 4

alternative NHS beds or to jointly plan alternative community-based provision. Thus, the proposed transfer of 750 patients (435 being over 60 years old) as a result of such a closure led to the comment that "it is in this vital area of community care which is still far from a practical reality that the hospital and the local authority need to combine forces and plan for the future"[5].

County Council (C) was calling for "nursing home type provision within the National Health Service for the more heavily dependent residents increasingly found in old people's homes"[6] as part of its response to the government's consultation paper on *A happier old age* (DHSS, 1978a). In 1983 it was addressing the much more specific issue of a closure of a long stay hospital for older people and its replacement with the use of 'new' beds at three community hospitals. Although supportive overall, the Social Services Committee complained that "these proposals were drawn up without involving the local authority"[7], given the resource implications for hospital social workers (the transfer of patients) and area teams (the delivery of domiciliary and other services).

Finally, the Metropolitan Authority was taking a similar line in the late 1980s about the closure of an old 77 bed geriatric hospital. It agreed "facilities were inadequate to enable a satisfactory quality of life to be enjoyed by patients" and called upon the Health Authority to develop at least some NHS replacement beds, as well as more rehabilitation services. It also expressed concern at "the knock-on effect of a reduction in hospital beds on community based services, including home care, meals on wheels, district nursing services and the laundry service"[8].

Social services authorities tended not to oppose this shift in emphasis from NHS long stay provision to care in the community. They saw this as inevitable since it was a central plank of government policy. A former Director from the London Borough reflected that there "was open acknowledgement that transfer was occurring as a matter of national policy as well as local practice" (interview with Director of Social Services [A], 1980-83). There was also often an agreement that such a policy offered the prospect of an improved quality of life for many vulnerable people, many of whom were older. Thus, a Director from County Council (B) commented that:

> ... [the] Chief Executive of the Local Health Authority ... was a real dynamo ... who had a passionate belief that all the old health institutions, primarily mental hospitals and geriatric hospitals were obsolete, too expensive, too many overheads and were full of people who didn't require

health care. So it was the same sort of belief that we had begun to feel.
(interview with Director of Social Services [B], 1971-90)

However, tensions arose over the failure either to transfer adequate
resources to social services or to develop alternative NHS based community
provision.

Such a situation encouraged in some of our respondents a cynical view
of the policy drive behind the reductions in 'continuing care' beds. It
was seen as a simple way to cut costs in a health service dominated by
acute care and the voracious need for resources for teaching hospitals. A
former local authority health visitor lamented that after the 1974 NHS
reorganisation "hospitals were ... all people ever thought of" (interview
with Health Visitor [D], 1971-87). More dramatically, a former Chief
Officer for a Community Health Council claimed that "if you've a teaching
hospital in your midst, it's like having a bloody great monster sucking the
blood from every other part" (interview with Chief Officer of Community
Health Council [C], 1977-93) of the local health service. He felt such a
situation often led to a complete failure to develop adequate community
health services. A Director of Social Services from the same area also
referred to the Health Authority as "teaching hospital dominated", leading
to "underinvestment in community nursing services" (interview with
Director of Social Services [C], 1988-95).

The London Borough opposed government proposals to change how
resources were allocated to health authorities since this would reduce the
budget of the Area Health Authority by between £9 million and £13
million. The new formula had been designed to achieve more equity of
resource distribution across the country, a strategy that required 'penalising'
those health authorities with high expenditure on teaching hospitals.
However, the Borough argued that "the financing of medical teaching
and research is, and should be regarded as an issue separate from the
financing of district health services"[9]. It argued that "cuts of this magnitude
would throw intolerable demands on the local social services and on
general practitioners"[10]. The assumption behind the quotation is that
cutbacks in community health services were a far more likely outcome
than the closure of one of the two teaching hospitals that were consuming
all the resources.

What is health care? What is social care?

Changes in the NHS that were impacting on social services provision for
older people were not limited to the reduction of long stay beds. By the

late 1970s and early 1980s the move towards quick patient turnover in hospitals was already being felt. A former Director of Social Services in the Metropolitan Authority referred to this as a trend towards "assessment … (and) short term treatment" (interview with Director of Social Services [D], 1977-87) in hospital backed up by support on discharge from community health services. This was not always seen as unproblematic by social services. For example, the 1977-86 consultative strategic plan for the Area Health Authority for the London Borough stressed that "the large district general hospitals are likely to become places more for the scientific and technological investigation of patients"[11] with community health services taking on much more of the responsibility for ongoing health and welfare support. The implications of all this for social services were a major concern and it was argued that it was "essential to have spelt out the condition of patients on discharge from acute hospital beds in order to know not only what care is needed but who is most appropriate to provide such care in the community"[12].

Such comments, and some of the other quotations already used, indicate how trends in the health service were causing tensions between health and social services. These tensions were often played out in terms of debates about 'what is health care?' and 'what is social care?', with social services often concerned that they were being asked to take on health service work with no additional resources. As one of the respondents from County Council (C) put it "Social Services feel that they've been, to coin a phrase 'dumped on' to a degree with a lot of what should have been and should continue to be health responsibility" (interview with Joint Commissioner [C], 1992-93).

These tensions and dumping concerns spanned both residential care and domiciliary services. In terms of the former, Chapter Four has already highlighted local authority worries about the increased dependency of residents. Typical of the links between reductions in NHS continuing care provision (plus the failure to develop appropriate alternative NHS provision) and the demand on residential care staff is the following 1977 quotation from County Council (C):

> Reference to Part III accommodation currently providing some type of nursing care graphically highlights the problems which are currently falling on the Social Services Department by providing services which are inappropriate to their skills and resources. These pressures will continue, and the Department and its staff will need to take great care that inappropriate burdens are not passed to them. However, they should be diminished if the Health Service develops facilities for the elderly[13].

The response from the NHS side to these types of concern was not always very sympathetic. For example, the London Borough had identical concerns to County Council (C) and these had been expressed in a report on growing dependency levels among residents (see previous chapter). However, the response of the Area Health Authority was to explain that these concerns reflected a failure to appreciate the redefinition of nursing that had taken place:

> In recalling ... the high level of nursing care needed by a significant number of residents, the Committee were informed of the changing nature of the definition of the term 'nursing care'. Dr 'X' explained how in the sphere of the Area Health Authority nursing was now being considered as part of the service which required very specialist skills rather than 'simply' caring[14].

Nevertheless, social services authorities, even when they accepted these changes, still felt unable to access adequate medical support for their frailest and sickest residents.

Indeed, this last concern was found in all four case studies. Thus, as early as 1972, County Council (B) was calling for improved GP liaison and consultant coverage for its own residential homes because of the changing health profile of residents[15]. In 1975, the concern of the London Borough was the need to access community nursing services to help with those residents with incontinence, severe confusion and/or a need for regular medication[16]. The Metropolitan Authority was worried about the very same issue in 1979 as a result of a survey of arrangements for medical care in local authority homes. Such medical care was deemed to be inadequate, leading to two main recommendations:

> A clinical medical officer should undertake geriatric screening of new admissions ... in order that remediable conditions be treated, appropriate placement achieved and unnecessary admissions avoided[17].

> The attachment of one district nurse to each home is recommended in order to achieve closer working relationships with care staff, for the benefit of residents[18].

Finally, County Council (C) was discussing in 1985 the need to improve the medical care of those residents who raised issues relating to "the management of problems of infirmity, drug control, incontinence, disability"[19].

The emphasis of the chapter has so far been on the impact on local authority residential care of reductions in NHS continuing care beds. However, it has already become clear that this is closely entwined with issues relating to the development (or non-development) of community health services, and how this in turn related to agreement (or non-agreement) about the respective roles and responsibilities of health and social services.

The widely held concern about the failure of the NHS to invest in community health services or to transfer significant resources to social services has already been noted. It was seen by some as a case of "closure of long stay hospital wards and only small increases in domiciliary health care"[20]. Even when bold new strategies were developed, social services were sometimes frustrated by the tendency to plan "on the basis of far more generous resource assumptions than those considered appropriate to the local authority"[21]. In other words, local authorities were expected to invest in new services beyond what councillors felt could realistically be made available. However, frustrations were not all one sided. The Health Authority was complaining in the early 1980s to social services in County Council (C) about the lack of availability of the home help service at weekends and the knock-on consequence of this in terms of increased workloads for district nurses[22].

The overall situation seemed to encourage tensions around roles and responsibilities related to differing definitions of 'what is health care?' and 'what is social care?' Such concerns were often played out in terms of day-to-day operational difficulties between health and social services staff because it was at that level "where all the frictions and abrasions occurred because of perceptions of being dumped upon" (interview with Director of Social Services [A], 1980-83). This former Director went on to explain how the closure of a bath attendant service run by the Health Authority generated numerous arguments among field level staff over the definition of a medical/nursing bath as opposed to a social one.

Such tensions were being generated by resource pressures on health as well as social services, resulting in a need for health to prioritise the work of primary health care workers. Thus, the respondent just quoted also noted how hard it was to agree on roles and responsibilities with health "because it's a moving target":

> Their resources were not going up. The demand was going up. And they in practice were therefore having to exclude people from their service who'd previously received health support and we were of course picking up demand which would have gone to them. So there was a

constant debate ... who were their patients and our clients. (interview
with Director of Social Services [A], 1980-83)

The resultant trends were profiled by County Council (C) in a report
that showed that the district nurse workload had dropped in terms of
patients, from 49,879 in 1984 to 25,539 in 1988/89. However, the number
of visits in the same period had risen from 326,432 to 465,972[23].

Day hospitals and day care was another area of frequent dispute and
disagreement. A residential services officer from County Council (B)
noted how day care was provided by health, the local authority and the
voluntary sector in the early 1970s. He remembered "how there was
great discussion as to who should provide the day care" (interview with
Residential Services Officer/Principal Officer, Registration Services [B],
1965-83). However, he had attended one meeting where a very simple
solution was proposed based on transport requirements:

> If you needed to be conveyed by ambulance you went to the hospital.
> If you could be conveyed by a minibus or by car with someone, then
> you would go to the day care centre, a staffed day care centre. Whereas
> if you could go by car or you were ambulant, you went to the day
> centre that was run by voluntary (organisations). (interview with
> Residential Services Officer/Principal Officer, Registration Services [B],
> 1965-83)

Such crude and simplistic approaches to targeting would struggle to survive
the harsh financial climate of the 1980s.

One reason for this was that from the perspective of health, many older
people were using day hospitals for essentially social rather than health
reasons. This was a finding of the visit of the Health Advisory Service
and the Social Work Service to County Council (C) in early 1981. Its
review of services for older people had found that some patients in day
hospitals were attending for social reasons and recommended to the Area
Health Authority that the criteria for attendance should be more strictly
defined, with those suitable for day centres being referred to the social
services department. The response of the latter was that "should this
advice be followed it would not be possible from within present resources
available to social services to provide those referred with places or the
level of care required"[24].

What were the main responses of social services to these ongoing debates
about how to define the boundary between health and social care? One
approach was to try and develop detailed protocols that set out the roles

and responsibilities of each, an approach tried in County Council (B) towards the end of the study period (interview with Chair, Social Services Committee [B], 1989-93). Indeed, at times definitional clarity on this point was seen as a mechanism by which inappropriately placed older people could be 'traded' between health and social services. Thus, one of the responses of the Metropolitan Authority to the *Care in the community* (DHSS, 1981b) consultative document in terms of the local situation was that:

> As far as the elderly are concerned, the situation is currently under investigation with the Area Health Authority. However, it would not be pre-empting any work to say that there are inevitably some people currently in hospital who could be discharged to local authority accommodation at present, but this could be offset by people receiving local authority services who really need hospital care[25].

The logic of protocols, rigid definitions and eligibility criteria is that they discourage the inappropriate placement of older people.

However, not all were convinced that this was the best way to tackle the issue. Some felt such definitional attempts were doomed to failure and that a much less formal style was required. A former Director of Social Services for the London Borough commented:

> My recollection … was that we would sit down and discuss what it was we wanted to achieve and whoever had the money that year funded it…. It was when you had to retreat and make the definition that it actually became problematic. (interview with Director of Social Services [A], 1986-94)

This approach suggested that it would never be possible to be completely clear about the boundary between health and social care. For some this was because of the extent of the overlap of the actual roles of workers such as home helps and nursing assistants. This had led the Residential and Day Services Officer in the Metropolitan Authority to propose "a single job description because there was a lot of scope for us to be working together much more closely" (interview with Residential and Day Services Manager/District Officer [D], 1985-93). He felt that there were genuine overlaps in roles and that a pooling of staff resources across health and social services would be a more constructive approach than arguing over who has responsibility for which clients. However, this suggestion was not taken up. It was seen as far too radical. Having said this, by March

1989 the same authority was beginning to discuss the feasibility of "joint planning of services with the health authority and voluntary organisations, including pooling of financial and other resources"[26]. Indeed, the main mechanism created by central government for overcoming boundary disputes was joint care planning and joint finance. However, these mechanisms could become a source of additional friction rather than a solution to boundary problems and interagency working.

Joint finance and joint planning

Although a full content analysis was not carried out on joint finance projects for the period of study, it was possible to identify some broad trends. In the early years of joint finance there were a number of schemes that supported local authorities as they attempted to cope with increased dependency levels in their residential homes. Many of these schemes were quite modest (for example, improved aids and more readily available adaptations), but others were more ambitious, such as the attempt by the Metropolitan Authority to establish a high dependency home aimed at those requiring "considerable caring and nursing but not medical treatment"[27]. The proposal was to use an existing local authority home and to introduce nursing staff (interview with Director of Social Services [D], 1987-93), together with a joint consultation mechanism on admissions and treatment/caring options between social services and local geriatricians. The initial contribution of the Area Health Authority was to be met through joint finance with an ongoing commitment from both health and social services to continue the scheme beyond the joint finance period. Although it took a considerable time to persuade the Health Authority to support the proposal (interview with General Secretary, Council of Voluntary Service/Chief Officer, Age Concern [D], 1973-81), the home was eventually established, although its initial impact was somewhat lessened by the delay in appointing a geriatrician[28]. Similar developments were found in County Council (C) where the problem became the high staffing costs of the two homes that were established (interview with Assistant Director of Social Services [C], 1978-83).

Joint finance was also used to help fund the kind of community services that social services often complained were absent yet essential, if the NHS was to reduce its provision of continuing care beds. The Metropolitan Authority developed a community laundry service with joint finance monies[29], the London Borough developed respite services[30], County Council (B) expanded its home care provision[31] and County Council (C) developed its day care provision[32]. One feature of the grants was that they were often used to develop the role of the voluntary sector in the provision of community-based services. Thus, County Council (C) grant aided a local Age Concern group to set up a lodgings scheme[33], while the Metropolitan Authority developed a Crossroads Care Attendant Scheme[34], which also involved using urban aid monies (see next chapter for more detail).

All of this activity was not without its tensions. All four authorities expressed concern, and sometimes anger, at the assumption that they would be in a position to pick up revenue costs once the period of joint finance had come to an end. This was especially true of County Council (B), which in October 1976 agreed the following resolutions:

• that the Health Authority be informed that the council regretfully can accept no responsibility for any part of the cost of this joint programme at present or for the foreseeable future;
• that any staff for this programme (after consultation with any union concerned) be appointed for a fixed period of three years only. If subsequently 100% of the costs continues to be funded by the Health Authority, then the staff could be offered a new appointment on a more permanent basis;
• that if, despite this, some cost still falls upon the County Council, programme committees be informed that no further allocation of resources be made to them in future years to cover the cost of this programme. [35]

Over five years later the same tensions were still there with the Council agreeing to pick up revenue costs after joint finance only on the grounds that "the Area Health Authority had agreed ... that expenditure on services currently provided for within the Social Services revenue budget to a total cost of £403,000 be submitted as new projects under Joint Financing in 1982/83"[36].

In a rather less aggressive way, the Metropolitan Authority talked of how the content of the programme would be driven by the capacity of the local authority to pick up revenue costs[37]. In other words, there was a danger that the emphasis in joint finance programmes would be on capital projects with minimal revenue implications. The complaint of the London Borough was more general in that it felt that "it would be wrong to commit finance immediately to any long term projects, whether capital or revenue, which would pre-empt decisions in later years on priorities"[38], although it did indicate that it would be willing to consider this once a long-term priority framework had been agreed with the

Health Authority. Underlying all of this was perhaps resentment by social services that, as one manager put it, "they (the health authorities) had the money" (interview with Deputy Director/Area Director of Social Services [B], 1971-89).

However, frustrations with joint finance and joint care planning were not limited to these financial details. They were seen by some as a smokescreen to cover up and deflect attention away from cutbacks in mainstream services (interview with Chief Officer for Age Concern [C1], 1981-93) and by others as simply marginal to the massive issues faced by health and social services (interview with Director of Social Services [A], 1971-80). The sums of money were relatively small compared to overall health and social care budgets. Joint care planning teams were often seen as just "talk shops and very little came out of them" (interview with Residential Services Officer/Principal Officer, Registration Services [B], 1965-83). In a similarly negative vein, a former Director of Age Concern in the London Borough spoke of how "joint planning (was) a joke really" in which "meetings ... got cancelled every five minutes" (interview with Director, Age Concern [A], 1990-93).

Dementia struggles

One group of older people who have always been likely to generate tensions between health and social services are older people with dementia, as traced by our earlier study (Means and Smith, 1998a). During the period 1971 to 1993, one of the major challenges facing health and social services remained how to develop coherent services for this group, who were often still referred to as the elderly mentally infirm (EMI) and about whom there was considerable concern in respect of the public expenditure implications of their rapidly rising numbers (Health Advisory Service, 1983). Long stay hospital closures often involved older people with dementia, and one of the biggest conflicts between health and social care was over respective responsibilities for this group.

People with dementia have an organic illness (Burns et al, 1997; Wilcock, 1990; WHO, 1992), but there is often little medical intervention available or appropriate and so their greatest need is for social support. A consequence of this in the study period was growing numbers of older people with dementia in local authority residential care. One response was to use joint care planning and joint finance to develop both institution and home-based services for this group. Nevertheless, at the end of the study period dementia care services often remained either an area of conflict between health and social services or an area where provision was of poor quality and low priority.

For example, a Director of Social Services from the London Borough felt that the authority had been quite progressive in the development of its own residential provision for this group, but felt overall that services for this group were not a high priority, while "psychiatric services" in one of the main teaching hospitals "were always problematic and weren't really improved when I left" (interview with Director of Social Services [A], 1986-94). County Council (B) was in the process of redefining several of its establishments as EMI homes during the late 1970s. However, the admission criteria still stressed that although "a degree of restlessness by day and night is acceptable", EMI homes were not appropriate for those prone to "persistent wandering or disorientation" or for those exhibiting "aggressive behaviour" which could amount to "disturbance in relation to other residents"[39]. The Committee report offered no guidance over how to define when a degree of restlessness shaded into persistent wandering. In the same year the lack of NHS day hospital provision led the Director of Social Services to state "this must undoubtedly be the area of most concern and maximum co-operation"[40] between health and social services. Despite this a Health Advisory Service report on services for people with mental health problems and older people with dementia in one of the health districts within County Council (B) in the early 1990s, still felt it necessary to call for "much great expenditure on mental health services (budget is substantially below the English County average)"[41].

The situation in County Council (C) was often even more fraught. In 1977, the Social Services Committee was informed of a crisis in NHS long-term care for older people that was so pronounced that "it is doubtful if the services that exist can survive much longer without total collapse"[42]. The report called for both a new psychogeriatric unit and new purpose-built homes, and yet four years later the same Committee was being faced with the following highly critical comments from the Health Advisory Service:

> The report begins by summarising main issues and these are that in the Health Service, because of economic stringencies and the financial implications of opening the X Hospital, the increasing demands of the elderly mentally infirm in particular have not been met and that this remains an outstanding problem with the lack of health provision causing very severe stress on community and residential social services[43].

Seven years on, major difficulties and tensions remained. The Health Authority had declared that "hospital care should not be regarded as a permanent home"[44] and that the service emphasis should switch to community teams and resource centres. Although happy with these principles, social services felt that far too much of the responsibility for future service development and provision was being left with them, without any additional resources. Hence, the Chief Executive of the local authority wrote to the District General Manager to complain that "the proposals in the Consultation Document involve a level of resource commitment from the County Council which they are unable to give at the moment"[45].

Health and social services also struggled in the Metropolitan Authority over this issue. As early as May 1976, a report from the Psychiatric Services Visiting Panel criticised the generally poor accommodation standards for all patients and the specific lack of designated beds or a unit for psychogeriatric patients, as well as calling for a more joint approach to planning by health and social services[46]. The local authority did produce a 30 page report on "services for confused elderly people"[47] in June 1983, which attempted to define the respective roles of health and social services, and which outlined proposed service developments by the local authority in excess of £500,000. However, the Health Advisory Service in its report on services for people with mental health problems and people with dementia in 1992 still criticised the lack of clear joint planning, despite the presence of joint care planning teams[48].

Working relationships: an overview

The emphasis in this chapter has so far been on day-to-day tensions and difficulties between health and social services. This final section takes a broader view of these relationships and draws mainly from interviews with key respondents.

It needs to be remembered that despite the problems, imaginative joint planning and joint projects did emerge. For example, a by-product of the critical review of mental health services in County Council (C) was a joint protocol on the management of disturbed behaviour[49]. The same authority also helped to pioneer joint commissioner posts between health and social services. Similar positive examples of joint working were found in all four case studies.

Indeed, senior social services managers amongst the respondents often painted a relatively positive view of relations between managers from both sides. Thus, a Director of Social Services for the London Borough spoke of the "extraordinary good working relationship with certainly the senior personnel, chief executives and so on in the Health Service" (interview with Director of Social Services [A], 1971-80). The next Director in the same authority indicated that "the relationship with health was a good one" (interview with Director of Social Services [A], 1980-83). A Deputy Director of Social Services from County Council (B) stated that the authority:

> ... seems to me to have always had a good working relationship with health across the board both at policy level, sort of in agreeing things that needed to be done and how staff will work together and actually staff working together. (interview with Deputy Director of Social Services [B], 1989-93)

This outlook was echoed by a Director of Social Services in the Metropolitan Authority who spoke of "an extraordinary good relationship of joint working" (interview with Director of Social Services [D], 1987-93). Not everyone, of course, was so sanguine. A Director of Social Services from County Council (C) felt that he had inherited "very poor relationships with a very powerful health service" (interview with Director of Social Services [C], 1988-95). A director from the London Borough felt that at times the local authority had too little control or influence over what the Health Service did (interview with Director of Social Services [A], 1986-94). Even among those with the most positive views, this was often tempered by considerable reservations. Thus, one of the directors from the London Borough may have said relations were good, but he also admitted that he might be "painting a little bit of a rosy picture because there was blood on the carpet from time to time, simply because of the sheer pressure" (interview with Director of Social Services [A], 1980-83). An Assistant Director from the Metropolitan Authority felt relations with health were good, but reflected that they were "of a traditional status quo kind rather than of a mutually challenging kind" (interview with Assistant Director of Social Services [D], 1977-87). On an equally self critical note, a former Deputy Director and then Director from County Council (B) stated that relations were good given the obstacles to joint working, but still felt "on a personal basis" that he should "have spent more time trying to be creative in the use of joint services" (interview with Deputy Director and Director of Social Services [B], 1971-90).

Both individual personalities and geographical boundaries were seen by many of the respondents as crucial to fostering or undermining good working relationships between health and social services. Thus, one Director of Social Services felt that strained working relationships with the Chief Executive of the Health Authority was a reflection of the fact that this individual "never really accepted that local authorities were in the lead in community care" (interview with Director of Social Services [A], 1986-94). This respondent also thought that the local authority had suffered in terms of working relationships with health after health reorganisation made it no longer coterminous with a single health authority. A similar type of comment was also made by a respondent from County Council (B) who pointed out that the lack of coterminosity had made it very difficult for social services to provide adequate representation on all the joint care planning teams of both health authorities (interview with Deputy Director/Area Director of Social Services [B], 1971-89). By way of contrast at an operational level, the decision of County Council (B) to implement a radical decentralisation of its social services was seen as fostering good joint working with primary care 'on the ground' (interview with Deputy Director and Director of Social Services [B], 1971-90).

Towards the end of the study period, social services authorities seemed to feel the need to 'get on' with health as an ever-greater strategic priority. The Director of Social Services for County Council (C) responded to the inheritance of poor relations with health in 1988 by instigating a monthly meeting between himself, the Chief Executive of the Health Authority and the Chief Executive of the Family Practitioner Committee. This was the three GMs (General Managers) meeting and "the three GMs meeting was monthly, coming together to pull the health and social services agenda together" (interview with Director of Social Services [C], 1988-95). In a similar yet more formal way, the Metropolitan Authority established a Joint Health Executive to be "the lead group to oversee the preparation for community care"[50]. Such moves were not always appreciated, with one Chief Executive of an Age Concern group in County Council (C) feeling that the inner sanctum of 'the three GMs meeting' froze out the voice of the voluntary sector (interview with Chief Officer, Age Concern [C1], 1981-93). The view of the Director of Social Services was rather different, feeling that he had learnt from bitter experience that the Health Authority had little sway over the NHS trusts, and policies agreed at these 'three GMs meetings' had often failed to get implemented (interview with Director of Social Services [C], 1988-95).

Conclusion

Boundaries between health and social care continued to shift throughout the study period, but they shifted mainly in one direction. Social services were expected to take on responsibilities for older people who would once have been deemed to lie well outside any definition of "in need of care and attention". Not only this but they were expected to work ever more closely with health over the planning and delivery of services, especially at the community level. The resultant tensions and arguments outlined in this chapter were perhaps inevitable. However, what is perhaps equally striking is how senior social services managers from the four case studies recognised both the problems faced by health and the need to find a way to work across the famous 'Berlin wall' divide (Dobson, 1997) between the two. The implications of this for the proposals of the Labour government to establish care trusts (Secretary of State for Health, 2000a, p 73) are discussed in the final chapter.

Notes

[1] Social Services Committee (A), 17 January 1977 ('X' Hospital).

[2] Social Services Committee (A), 27 January 1982 (Transfer of Patients).

[3] Social Services Committee (B), 7 June 1971 (Quarterly Report of the Director of Social Services).

[4] Social Services Committee (B), 21 September 1978 (Strategy for Health in the 1990s).

[5] Social Services Committee (B), 4 July 1972 (After Hospital – What Next?).

[6] Social Services Committee (C), 8 December 1978 (A Happier Old Age – A Discussion Document on Elderly People in our Society).

[7] Social Services Committee (C), October 1983 (Care of the Elderly – New Community Beds: A Consultative Document).

[8] Social Services Committee (D), 2 August 1988 (Closure of Hospital).

[9] Social Services Committee (A), 17 January 1977 (Sharing Resources for Health in England – Report of the Resource Allocation Working Party).

[10] Ibid.

[11] Social Services Committee (A), 1 May 1977 (Consultative Area Strategic Plan 1977-86: Commentary by the Community Care Programme Group).

[12] Ibid.

[13] Social Services Committee (C), 18 March 1977 (Area Health Authority [Teaching] – Creation of First Health Area Plan).

[14] Social Services Committee (A), 22 November 1976 (Elderly, Physically Handicapped and Ill, and Community Development Review Committee).

[15] Social Services Committee (B), 6 December 1972 (Medical Survey in Homes for the Elderly).

[16] Social Services Committee (A), 8 December 1975 (Dependency Levels of Residents in Council Homes for Elderly People).

[17] Social Services Committee (D), 5 June 1979 (Residential Homes for the Elderly: Arrangements for Medical Care).

[18] Ibid.

[19] Social Services Committee (C), 7 June 1985 (Medical Services in Old People's Homes).

[20] Health Authority Consultation Document (C), October 1983 (Care of the Elderly – New Community Beds).

[21] Social Services Committee (C), 8 June 1984 (Health Authority: Draft Strategic Plan).

[22] Social Services Committee (C), 11 September 1981 (Commentary by the Director of Social Services on a Report of a Visit by the Health Advisory Service and Social Work Service of the DHSS).

[23] Social Services Committee (C), 30 November 1989 (Review of Current Services for Elderly People).

[24] Social Services Committee (C), 11 September 1981 (Commentary by the Director of Social Services on a Report of a Visit by the Health Advisory Service and Social Work Service of the DHSS).

[25] Social Services Committee (D), 29 September 1981 (Comments on Care in the Community).

[26] Social Services Committee (D), 21 March 1989 (Development of Services for Elderly People).

[27] Social Services Committee (D), 3 August 1976 (Report on DHSS Circular on Joint Care Planning).

[28] Social Services Committee (D), June 1976 (Joint High Dependency Home).

[29] Joint Consultative Committee (D), 23 January 1976 (Domiciliary Laundry Service).

[30] Social Services Committee (A), 31 January 1989 (Respite Care for Elderly People).

[31] Social Services Committee (B), 26 October 1976 (Joint Care Planning, Health and Local Authorities).

[32] Social Services Committee (C), 9 September 1977 (Joint Finance 1977-78: Day Centre).

[33] Social Services Committee (C), 9 September 1977 (Report of the Joint Care Planning Team).

[34] Social Services Committee (D), 9 June 1981 (Implications for the Council's Services of the Area Health Authority's Operational Plan, 1981-84).

[35] Social Services Committee (B), 26 October 1976 (Joint Care Planning – Health and Local Authorities).

[36] Social Services Committee (B), 22 April 1982 (Joint Consultative Committee).

[37] Joint Consultative Committee (D), 25 June 1976 (Joint Care Planning – Health and Local Authorities).

[38] Social Services Committee (A), 27 September 1976 (Joint Finance).

[39] Social Services Committee (B), 9 June 1978 (Elderly Mentally Infirm Provision).

[40] Social Services Committee (B), September 1978 (Strategy for Health in the 1980s).

[41] Social Services Committee (B), 19 September 1991 (Report on Services for Mentally Ill People and Elderly People).

[42] Social Services Committee (C), 18 March 1977 (Care of the Elderly Mentally Infirm).

[43] Social Services Committee (C), 11 September 1981 (Commentary of Director of Social Services on a Report of a Visit by the Health Advisory Service of the DHSS).

[44] Social Services Committee (C), 27 July 1988 (Mental Health Consultation Document).

[45] Ibid.

[46] Joint Consultative Committee (D), 21 May 1976 (Interim Report of the Psychiatric Services Visiting Panel).

[47] Social Services Committee (D), 17 June 1983 (Services for Confused Elderly People).

[48] Joint Health Executive (D), 7 September 1992.

[49] Social Services Committee (C), 5 March 1991 (Disturbed Behaviour in Elderly People).

[50] Social Services Committee (D), 14 January 1991 (Preparation for Community Care).

SIX

Towards a mixed economy of social care for older people?

Introduction

One of the strongest policy themes of successive Conservative governments during the study period was a dislike and a suspicion of the local authority as the dominant provider of welfare services (Means and Smith, 1998b). They were perceived as expensive and unresponsive to the needs of the consumer. Welfare pluralism (Johnson, 1987) or the mixed economy of social care (Wistow et al, 1994) was seen as offering a much more fruitful way forward. Reactions to this perspective were varied with concerns expressed about both the use of the private sector as a service provider (Langan, 1990) and about the potential loss of autonomy of the voluntary sector as a result of a move towards a contract culture (Deakin, 1996; Lewis, 1993). At the same time, there was also recognition of the possibilities created by the mixed economy, as emphasised by Taylor and Hoggett (1994, p 185):

> The opportunity exists to develop a diversity of provision catering for a range of different needs and preferences. Voluntary and private organisations as well as the consumers they serve should be in a position to gain a great deal from such a move. Indeed these are the kinds of policies which key thinkers on the voluntary sector were advocating back in the 1970s. (Hadley and Hatch, 1981; Wolfenden Committee, 1978)

This chapter explores the development of the mixed economy in services for older people in the four local authorities and specifically how the role of the voluntary sector changed during the study period. However, the chapter begins by commenting on the already changing role of voluntary organisations involved with older people during the 1960s.

The voluntary sector and older people in the 1960s

In their previous study, the authors profiled the changing role of the voluntary sector in the provision of welfare services for older people from 1939 to 1971 (Means and Smith, 1998a). During the Second World War, voluntary organisations such as the British Red Cross Society, the National Old People's Welfare Committee (NOPWC) (now Age Concern) and the Women's (Royal) Voluntary Service (WRVS) developed a range of innovative services such as small residential homes, meals on wheels, luncheon clubs and visiting services. They were keen to further develop such activities after the war and they were supported in this aspiration by Beveridge (1948) who argued that the welfare state reforms of the 1940s should not be allowed to reduce the scope for voluntary action.

The 1948 National Assistance Act gave local authorities the lead role in the provision of residential care, but only very prescribed powers for narrowly defined groups of disabled people with regard to domiciliary services. For example, local authorities were not allowed to run their own meals services and were given no general powers to provide preventative services. This was partly a reflection of the desire to retain a clear role for the voluntary sector, but also reflected pessimism from senior civil servants at the Ministry of Health about the potential of domiciliary services to stop older people entering residential care. In other words, they were seen as an extra frill to be provided by voluntary organisations for the lonely and temporarily ill who lacked family support (Means and Smith, 1998a).

In 1948-49 Labour authorities such as Liverpool, York and Blackburn were pressing for permission to develop visiting services for older people in their own homes. In April 1949, Barbara Castle (then MP for Blackburn) asked the Minister of Health (Aneurin Bevan) if the 1948 Act could be interpreted as legalising such services and he agreed to look into this. However, civil service advice to the minister was that "the job is essentially one for voluntary rather than local authority effort" (quoted in Means and Smith, 1998a, p 140).

The subsequent circular on the *Welfare of old people* argued that the experience gained since 1948:

> ... has shown an urgent need for further services of the more personal kind which are not covered by existing statutory provision and which indeed are probably best provided by voluntary workers activated by a spirit of good neighbourliness. (MoH, 1950)

Local old people's welfare committees were asked to coordinate such effort. As has been argued elsewhere, "this circular is often described as representing a liberalisation of government policy when really it was an attempt to ensure local authorities remained focused narrowly upon the provision of residential care" (Means, 1993, p 159).

As discussed in earlier chapters, such a consensus did not last. The emphasis on local authority residential care was undermined by the research by Townsend (1962) and others. At the same time, local authorities were becoming frustrated at the failure of voluntary organisations to develop coherent authority-wide provision of services in areas such as meals on wheels, day care and visiting/counselling schemes. This created what one commentator of the time called a "wind of discontent" in town halls (Slack, 1960). Voluntary organisations such as NOPWC and WRVS were tending to argue amongst themselves about how to coordinate services. Volunteer availability was varied, with recruitment often easiest in areas with the least need. Services were not only patchy, but where they did exist they often ran for only a few days a week and closed during school holidays (Means and Smith, 1998a, Chapter Six).

The full legal powers for local authorities to provide domiciliary services for older people did not occur until 1971, the start of our study period. A 1962 amendment of the 1948 National Assistance Act enabled local authorities to provide and deliver their own meals on wheels services. The 1968 Health Services and Public Health Act made it mandatory for local authorities to run a home help service (previously this was just a permissive power) and gave them a general power to promote the welfare of older people. The 1970 Chronically Sick and Disabled Persons Act placed a further set of obligations on local authorities (for example, assessment for telephones and home adaptations), although the implementation of this and the 1968 Act was delayed to coincide with the introduction of unified social services departments in April 1971.

The traditional voluntary sector and older people

Despite this wind of discontent and the expansionist environment for local authorities in the early 1970s (see Chapters Three and Four), all the case study authorities continued to stress the important role of the voluntary sector. Thus, the London Borough in a review of the 1968 Act noted how:

> Voluntary organisations and voluntary workers have an indispensable
> part to play in service for the elderly. A social basis of support from the

local authority professional staff is essential; but both because of the special contribution of flexibility, independence and informality which voluntary work can bring, and because of the scarcity of manpower both skilled and unskilled, development must depend very substantially on the help of volunteers[1].

In a similar vein, County Council (B) was talking of the need "to provide increasing opportunities for voluntary organisations and individuals to initiate, supplement and extend the Council's own services"[2]. Similar examples were found in the other two case studies.

Typical examples of this type of voluntary work were lunch clubs and social clubs for older people as well as meals on wheels services. Lunch clubs and social clubs were common in all four authorities and many of them were completely dependent on volunteer help. Thus one Over 60s Club met in the London Borough on Tuesday afternoons from 2-4pm[3]. It was run by a volunteer club leader and in 1982 had an annual turnover of just over £1,000 of which the bulk was member payments and only £190 was a grant from the local authority. The Metropolitan Authority was perhaps the most enthusiastic supporter of such clubs, seeing them as a crucial preventative deterrent against isolation[4], and by 1980 it had 32 luncheon clubs and a further 60 local day centres[5]. Local clubs in this authority were supported by voluntary services officers employed by the local authority[6], while in the two county case studies (B and C), this was seen as very much a key role for the secretaries/chief officers/directors of local Age Concern groups (interview with Director Age Concern [B], 1971-93). A report on such provision in the Metropolitan Authority as late as 1980 noted how "many of the 'volunteers' were themselves elderly, some luncheon clubs being run virtually on a self-help basis"[7].

Local authorities debated whether such clubs should be supported on the grounds of their very general preventative contribution in which they were seen as a 'good thing' for more active older people, or whether the work of the clubs should be encouraged to become more focused on those older people more likely to be at risk of residential care entry. And if services needed to be targeted at priority groups, was the local authority or the voluntary sector best placed to run such a service? Could volunteers and the voluntary sector provide a reliable service? These debates were especially fierce over meals on wheels services. Views varied, both between case studies and over time.

At the beginning of the study period three of the case studies (the two County Councils and the Metropolitan Authority) were completely dependent on the WRVS and its volunteers for the provision of meals services, and all three were to go through a process of reviewing whether this could be allowed to continue. The exception to this was the London Borough where all meals were delivered by local authority staff. This may have partly been a reflection of the fact that meals on wheels were seen by this authority as a core service and were the sole responsibility of the local authority. However, it may also have been due to the fact that the WRVS had struggled for a long time to maintain sufficient volunteers to run services in many larger urban conurbations (Harris, 1961; Slack, 1960).

County Council (B) also encountered a shortage of volunteers by the late 1970s. Initially, the largest city in the County was moving to local authority vans and drivers because "the WRVS had difficulty covering the service" (interview with Deputy Director/Area Director of Social Services [B] 1971-1989). However, by 1978, it was still a service largely dependent on the WRVS, as illustrated by Table 6.1. However, Table 6.1 also illustrates that the service tended to be available on only two or possibly three days per week when run solely by the WRVS, but was much more likely to be a five days per week service when the local authority was directly involved. By the mid-1980s, the local authority was reviewing this service and concluded that two main changes were needed. The first of these was to move towards frozen foods produced

Table 6.1: Organisations in County Council (B) providing meals 6/12 November 1978[8] (number of days per week to older people)

Number of days per week	Number of older people being supplied with meals				
	Local authority (LA)	Women's Royal Voluntary Service	Joint WRVS and LA	Total Number	%
1	4	113	4	121	3.1
2	60	2,069	26	2,155	55.0
3	69	764	31	864	22.1
4	34	152	20	206	5.3
5	134	369	66	569	14.5
6	–	1	–	1	–
7	–	1	–	1	–
Total	301	3,469	147	3,917	100.00

from distribution centres and away from reliance on a wide variety of small kitchens. The second was the need "to provide a comprehensive five day a week service, enhanced by the provision of meals on a seven day week basis for those clients in need of that support"[9]. The almost inevitable consequence of this decision was that the local authority gradually took over responsibility for both transport and driving (interview with Deputy Director/Area Director of Social Services [B], 1971-89), while the WRVS withdrew from food production. Their final withdrawal occurred in 1991, by which time the whole meals on wheels service (food, transport and delivery) had been contracted out to a 'for profit' organisation[10].

It was in the late 1970s that County Council (C) began to query whether it could continue to rely on the volunteers of the WRVS in order to deliver meals on wheels. This was driven from a desire to establish "a uniform pattern of provision throughout the County"[11], rather than a situation of a maximum of a few days per week service in most rural areas (WRVS run) compared to a five day per week service in the main urban area (jointly run by the WRVS, Red Cross and the local authority). However, the proposed way forward was not increased local authority input, but rather "extending the use made of voluntary organisations in taking responsibility for the provision of meals on wheels throughout the County"[12], although this was to be balanced by the local authority taking control over the referral process.

However, this was not to prove a long-term solution. Social services remained frustrated at the inability of the WRVS to extend its service to more days per week together with continuing meal availability problems on bank and school holidays (interview with Principal Officer (Elderly), Social Services [C], 1989-93). The WRVS also struggled to maintain volunteer coverage, as one former volunteer recalled:

> ... so I was filling in for people who were on holiday ... I can vividly remember one morning. I suddenly had a call at ten o'clock. Mrs So and So's car has broken down, can you possibly do a round this morning otherwise I'm up the creek sort of thing. And I was able to do it. (interview with Member and Chair of Pensioner's Action Group [C], 1985-93)

Relations were further strained over the quality of the food delivered. A survey indicated that it was little better than "soggy cardboard" (interview with Director of Social Services [C], 1988-95) and a decision was made to move to frozen foods, much to the chagrin of the WRVS.

A former Director of Social Services remembered how the combination of volunteer reliability and food quality led to "endless running battles … about meals on wheels … in which this nasty director … was seen as wrecking the WRVS" (interview with Director of Social Services [C], 1988-95). The impact of the introduction of frozen food on the meals on wheels service was considerable. It meant most older people could heat up their food as and when they wanted it and this "drastically cut the (meals on wheels) service" (interview with WRVS Organiser [C], 1992-93). However, the WRVS did not withdraw completely and indeed beyond the study period were to win the local authority contract to deliver meals across the County (interview with WRVS Organiser [C], 1992-93).

The WRVS played an even stronger role in the Metropolitan Authority being the sole deliverer of meals as late as 1980[13], as well as running a shopping service for housebound older people[14]. However, tensions were emerging over the capacity of the WRVS to provide a seven day a week service. The conclusion of the local authority was that they were not capable of doing this and so it was faced with the dilemma of how do you "expand … without upsetting them and inhibiting the volunteer spirit which you want to maintain" (interview with Director of Social Services [D], 1977-87). The other challenge, as with County Council (C), was the desire to introduce frozen and vacuum-packed food and to phase out the use of traditional kitchens. In the end, the late 1980s saw the launch of "a seven day meals on wheels service" in which the "WRVS did it during the week and the local authority did it in the evenings and at the weekend" (interview with Director of Social Services [D], 1987-93). However, a senior manager remembered how the need to close "most of the old kitchens" really did upset some of "the WRVS ladies" (interview with Director of Social Services [D], 1987-93).

If the WRVS was a significant player in three of our authorities, Age Concern groups featured strongly in all four of the case studies, although their emergence in some areas was much later than in others. Before these developments are profiled, it is necessary to say something about the constitution of local groups and their relationship to Age Concern (England). From its inception in 1971, the regulations of Age Concern (England) have included mechanisms by which locality-based charities can be formally recognised as Age Concern organisations. In other words, they are independent voluntary agencies that are allowed to use the term Age Concern in their title through meeting the criteria of membership of the National Council on Ageing. Under the present constitution, such organisations normally cover a population of around 75,000 and provide the basic functions of (i) services and support; (ii) public education and social advocacy; (iii) innovation and research; and (iv) partnership and cooperation. A further responsibility of such organisations since the early 1970s has been communication with and stimulation of more informal and localised Age Concern groups, some of which might go on to become Age Concern organisations in their own right.

The Metropolitan Authority gave strong support to its local Age Concern and was making grants to that organisation from the mid-1970s[15]. Age Concern (D) was created from the five old people's welfare committees that existed prior to the 1974 reorganisation of local authorities. The then General Secretary of the local Council of Voluntary Service (CVS) had played a pivotal role in a strategic review of services for older people[16] and was the driving force behind the establishment of Age Concern (D). However, Age Concern (D) in the 1970s remained part of the CVS and was not a legally constituted organisation in its own right (interview with General Secretary, Council of Voluntary Service [D], 1971-81).

Age Concern (D) did develop services in the 1970s such as welfare rights and information services, neighbourhood visiting schemes and day sitting services as well as developing in partnership with the local authority a major pop-in/day centre facility in the centre of the town (interview with General Secretary, Council of Voluntary Service [D], 1971-81, and with Director of Social Services [D], 1987-93). However, this was not seen as the central rationale for the organisation in this period:

> ... we provided services but only to give us the credibility to be able to bitch like crazy about the way social services, health, the government, whoever, was actually doing their job. And that fitted in with the framework of the Age Concern movement ... which (was) ... about education and advocacy. If you can't do those then you may as well call yourself WRVS or British Red Cross. (interview with General Secretary, Council of Voluntary Service [D], 1971-81)

However, nearly all of the work of Age Concern (D) was funded through the local authority and this caused one social services respondent to remark cynically that this made it very difficult for such organisations to have a genuinely independent voice (interview with Residential and Day Services Officer, District Officer [D], 1985-93).

County Council (C) had two long established Age Concerns[17]. Age Concern (C1) took the name of the County and covered all of the County, apart from the county town, which was covered by Age Concern (C2).

Initially Age Concern (C1) used to receive the whole Age Concern grant for the County but passed on 25% of the grant to help fund the part-time organiser for Age Concern (C2). However, Age Concern (C2) expanded to a point in the early 1980s where it had its own full-time organiser and made grant applications in its own right (interview with Organising Secretary/Chief Officer, Age Concern [C1], 1981-93, and with Organising Secretary Age Concern [C2], 1971-80).

Despite the emphasis of both Age Concerns on fundraising through charity shops and other mechanisms (interview with Organising Secretary, Age Concern [C2], 1971-80), grant aid to Age Concern from the local authority was considerable, reaching over £9,000 as early as 1977[18]. This money was used primarily to fund the organising secretaries whose role was very much to encourage volunteers to work with the fairly active older people, rather than to provide community care services. Age Concern (C2) did run a visiting service in the early 1970s and later developed five luncheon clubs/day centres[19]. Age Concern (C1) put an emphasis on voluntary field officers to offer support for older people in the villages and this especially involved "supporting clubs (for) ... the really active elderly"[20]. Age Concern (C1) received a joint finance grant to run an occasional day centre in one of the larger villages, but this was closed down at the end of the initial grant period[21]. The Organising Secretary felt that the emphasis was on "the summer sale and handicrafts exhibition" with "a committee to look after all sorts of trivial things" (interview with Organising Secretary/Chief Officer Age Concern [C1], 1981-93).

Joint planning, joint finance and joint care planning teams (see previous chapter) represented a crucial opportunity for this individual to escape the limitations of these roles. Both social services and the health authority needed to consult with the voluntary sector and Age Concern (C1) was keen to perform this role in relation to older people and to involve itself in all the new planning mechanisms (interview with Organising Secretary/ Chief Officer Age Concern [C1], 1981-93). Indeed, the Organising Secretary/Chief Officer became Chair of the Joint Consultative Committee for a period. The voluntary sector used such mechanisms to campaign around a number of controversial issues in County Council (C), including the introduction of increased charges for home care and day care, and the proposed closure of local authority residential homes (interview with Organising Secretary/Chief Officer Age Concern [C1], 1981-93, and with Organising Secretary, Age Concern [C2], 1971-80).

In County Council (B), the existing Old People's Welfare Committee received grants from 1971 to 1974 from a national charitable foundation to fund an organising secretary. In 1974, the Social Services Committee took over funding responsibility with a grant of £5,000 and the same officer continued the organising role in what by then had become Age Concern (B)[22]. This money effectively became the annual grant justified by an initial brief from Age Concern (B), which was "to research the needs of older people throughout the county and to meet those needs in whatever way appropriate, working alongside the seven district social services and the area health authority"[23]. The emphasis of the work was on developing separate Age Concern groups, several of which became formal Age Concern organisations in their own right (interview with Organising Secretary/Director of Age Concern [B], 1971-93).

The 1991/92 annual report noted how:

> Over the years, eleven local Age Concern groups have been inaugurated and the three former County Borough Age Concerns were assisted in becoming independent from the Councils of Voluntary Service. Fifty-four day centre or luncheon clubs have been established and innumerable social clubs. Age Concern (B) has acted as a resource for any agency or local Age Concern as and when required, supplied advice and information, arranged seminars, working parties and arranged conferences[24].

Although Age Concern (B) did run a respite and hospital aftercare service based on volunteer sitters, the emphasis of its work was on coordinating activity and encouraging the development of local voluntary organisations and groups across the County. This was in contrast to some of the newer Age Concern groups within the County where there was greater emphasis on service delivery[25]. As one respondent noted, local Age Concern groups often started out by running clubs but by the early 1990s were much more likely to be running a day centre for people with Alzheimer's disease on contract to the local authority (interview with Deputy Director/Area Director of Social Services [B], 1971-89, also interview with Academic [B], 1970-ongoing).

Criticism was also emerging from both local Age Concern groups and other local voluntary organisations towards Age Concern (B). Age Concern (B) was getting the largest grant of any voluntary organisation in the County (interview with Deputy Director and Director of Social Services [B], 1971-90), and these local groups felt they obtained very little practical support as a result. Social services began to share this criticism by the late 1980s on the grounds that "it was very difficult to know what they did and when they actually said what they did it couldn't be justified ... at all" (interview with Deputy Director of Social Services

[B], 1989-93). Financial pressures on local authorities were beginning to lead to a review of traditional ways of working with the voluntary sector (see below).

The London Borough developed a local Age Concern organisation much later than the other case studies. In the early 1980s the local authority funded an Age Concern Development Officer, which led to a fully independent Age Concern group from September 1982[26]. The new organisation focused in particular on developing a free newspaper, running an insurance service and campaigning on behalf of older people (interview with Chief Officer, Age Concern [A], 1982-83), rather than on providing community care services. The first Chief Officer remembered a service provider role being rejected by her committee, so even attempts to open lunch clubs or drop in day centres "were hampered by our committee", a view that was confirmed by two of the councillors who sat on the committee (interview with Chief Officer, Age Concern [A], 1982-83). In the early 1990s such attitudes had eased and the then Director was able to work with the local branch of the Alzheimer's Disease Society to open a day centre for people with dementia that was funded by the local authority as a major mixed economy initiative[27].

The growth of independent residential and nursing homes

Although the story of changing relationships between the traditional voluntary sector and local authorities is fascinating, the biggest impact on the mixed economy of social care was the rapid development of the independent residential and nursing home sector in the 1980s. This growth has already been noted in Chapter Four, which concentrated on the implications of this growth for the changing role of local authority residential care.

Three of the four case study authorities had only small private and voluntary homes prior to the 1980s. Thus, County Council (C) had 38 beds in voluntary residential homes in June 1971[28]. Although some local authorities placed older people in such homes, it was far less common to place people in private homes. As one social services respondent from the Metropolitan Authority remembered:

> There was a complete separation between public and private provision. So very small private provision in terms of numbers, very small, and in fact there was no overlap at all in the sense that ... you either were in

the private sector if you paid or you weren't. (interview with Director
of Social Services [D], 1977-87)

In the 1970s the focus of social services authorities in terms of residential
care was very much local authority provision.

Chapter Four outlined the sudden and massive expansion of both private
residential and nursing homes in the mid-1980s, described by one
respondent as "the unseen revolution" (interview with Social Worker/
Academic [B], 1971-93) and by another as "a monster" (interview with
Director of Social Services [D], 1977-87). This revolution was funded by
social security payments so large that one former Assistant Director of
Social Services spoke of how "the jaw drops open at the generosity"
(interview with Assistant Director of Social Services [D], 1977-87).
However, this 'monster' did not always lead to immediate conflict and
tension with the local authority. In County Council (C), a social services
respondent remembered how "there wasn't a kind of big antipathy between
the sectors, you know, they were just parallel sectors" (interview with
Deputy Director of Social Services [C], 1983-91).

In County Council (B) the Chair of the Private Residential Care Homes
Association remembers "a very good working relationship" with the local
authority prior to April 1993 (interview with Chair, Private Residential
Care Association [B], 1985-93).

However, tensions were beginning to build up as the 1980s progressed
as many local authorities came to terms with "having a residential home
on every street corner" (interview with Director of Social Services [D],
1987-93). Chapter Four focused on one aspect of this, namely the
implications for local authority residential care. As was seen, the transfer
of local authority homes was a popular option for many since it seemed
to open up the prospect of accessing social security benefits for highly
dependent social services clients. This often seemed more attractive than
refurbishing homes to meet new registration standards (too expensive) or
home closure (often politically unacceptable).

In areas such as County Council (B) where private provision was
extensive, the sector attempted early on to persuade the local authority
to concentrate on using private beds. However, this was not always well
received:

> ... because ... very early on there was this colossal boom in the private
> residential sector and they were clearly looking to the local authority
> to fill their beds and make them economically viable.... It was said
> that the traditional attitude of people in the statutory agencies towards

> people who were in it for profit really blinkered us ... to some of the
> opportunities that were presented by the fact that there were so many
> potentially new and valuable resources in the community. (interview
> with Deputy Director and Director of Social Services [B], 1972-90)

However, some respondents from the same authority reflected that the
obstacles to partnership working were not just a dislike of 'for profit'
organisations. It was also anger at their impact on employment conditions
in this sector. As one respondent put it, "what was obvious was that ...
the conditions and pay of our people were miles in advance of what ...
the private sector can get away with" (interview with Deputy Director
of Social Services [B], 1989-93). Not everyone saw this as a good example
of the efficiency of the market. The implications for low paid care staff
was one reason why Labour councillors, trades unions and others fought
proposed home closures in County Council (B) with such bitterness (see
Chapter Four).

In the late 1980s, many local authorities discovered a politically
acceptable way to close at least some of their homes and also to access
social security payments. This took the form of developing residential
and/or nursing home schemes in collaboration with 'not for profit'
voluntary organisations (and especially housing associations), rather than
with the private sector. New developments could thus be presented as
replacements rather than closure:

> That was a very specific but very major initiative to say the local
> authority's got some homes which aren't very good anymore. We will
> work with the voluntary sector to develop a replacement which will
> become an independent sector provision. (interview with Deputy
> Director of Social Services [C], 1983-91)

A slightly different approach, as seen in Chapter Four, was to try and
'float off' the local authority's residential homes under voluntary sector
management. However, this often foundered on the problem of the size
of the capital investment required to bring them up to registration standard.
Hence, the replacement approach became very popular in numerous local
authorities. This was very much the case in County Council (C). Thus,
in March 1991, the Social Services Committee approved a sheltered
housing with care scheme to be developed by a housing association "to
replace lost places resulting from the closure of homes" and to provide
"levels of care ... in individual flats equivalent to traditional residential

care"[29]. A report later in the same year outlined six such contracts with housing associations and another four were being proposed[30].

Sheltered housing with care schemes developed in this way usually involved social services having 100% nomination rights. They would put forward people who would otherwise go into local authority homes or be placed with the private sector (Means, 1999). For some in County Council (C), these schemes represented a "vision" (interview with Director of Social Services [C], 1988-95) of a more homely provision for highly dependent people, as well as a major stimulus to the development of the mixed economy of social care. However, not everyone was convinced:

> ... we were driven to an extremely expensive bed for bed replacement programme. So what we had to say because of the tremendous political flak ... 'we will replace every bed by direct fully funded provision. Here is a home, we regret we're going to close it. However, here around the corner is a lovely new flat, you know, twice as good ... your own space'.... And that was the selling point. (interview with Principal Officer (Elderly), Social Services [C], 1989-93)

This respondent felt that such an approach was flawed because the schemes proved very expensive to develop and deflected money away from investment in community support services. Older people were not always happy to be nominated because they "want to live in the closest home to their relatives ... and not in the home that you tell them that you happen to have built for them" (interview with Principal Officer (Elderly), Social Services [C], 1989-93).

One reason for the enthusiasm for joint schemes with housing associations was that they were a mechanism to develop the mixed economy as required by the Conservative government (interview with Principal Officer (Elderly), Social Services [C], 1989-93), but in a way acceptable to those Labour and Liberal Democrat councillors who were suspicious of, or hostile to, the private sector. The need to develop a mixed economy heightened as local authorities prepared for the 1 April 1993 community care changes in the knowledge that 85% of their social security transfer and transitional arrangement monies would need to go on funding services in the independent sector (Local Authority Social Services Letter 92/12, quoted in Lewis and Glennerster, 1996, p 31). Although the London Borough remained committed to local authority provided residential care, the guidelines meant that it needed a strategy for stimulating and supporting some independent provision in the post April 1993 system. It decided that of the 140-50 places it had wanted to purchase from this sector in 1993/94, 40% would be block purchased from the 10 most often used by local residents (nine of them in neighbouring boroughs) and 60% would be spot purchased from an approved list of 150 homes[31].

The issue in County Council (B) in the early 1990s was not the shortage of places in the private sector but the surplus. Transferred money to the local authority under the 1990 Act was cash limited and no longer ring fenced to residential/nursing home provision.

> We were cash limited. That's what the government wanted us to do, it was to stop the spiral of expenditure, so in 'B' you had a growing residential market, a huge market which was still growing, with a reduced budget. There was bound to be a squeeze. (interview with Director of Social Services [B], 1990-93)

Such a squeeze was certain to create tensions and arguments, because the private sector was in a contracting market:

> And that was worrying them. And we were still seen as ... being in the business and therefore by definition, we were going to be unfair and look after ourselves. (interview with Director of Social Services [B], 1990-93)

The private sector lobbied ministers in the Conservative government about this. The government in turn put pressure on the local authority (interview with Director of Social Services [B], 1990-93).

A former Chair of the Social Services Committee had considerable sympathy with the private sector over this, especially in terms of the desire of many homes to diversify into day care:

> Well, private homes ... [were] trying to put day centres on their premises. They haven't got any subsidy. They've got to borrow to do this and to my mind I don't think it's the business of a local authority to use public resources to subsidise their own services in competition with the private sector. (interview with Chair, Social Services Committee [B], 1989-93)

Despite this, some homes did diversify their activities. For example, the Chair of the Private Residential Care Homes Association said of his own home:

> We remain full, but I'm sure we wouldn't be if we'd stayed just elderly.
> We also diversified to the extent that we started doing meals on wheels
> ... which meant that we had contact with people out there. We also
> did respite care and day care. (interview with Chair, Private Residential
> Care Homes Association [B], 1980-93)

However, overall the then Director of Social Services in County Council
(B) felt the private sector was "slow to diversify" in response to the
community care changes and rather complacently assumed that existing
residential and nursing home care provision would carry on being
underpinned "with unlimited resources" (interview with Director of Social
Services [B], 1990-93).

If the private residential sector was slow to diversify into the development
of new service provision in the community, specialist private sector
suppliers of domiciliary care were beginning to emerge in County
Councils (B) (interview with Director of Social Services [B], 1990-93)
and (C)[32], driven by those older people who could pay for their own
support needs (cleaning, meals, personal support, and so on) without
recourse to social services.

Time limited grants, new service provision in the community and the voluntary sector

Before 1993, social services often looked to the voluntary sector to drive
new service developments and these were often funded by time-limited
grants. It seemed that local authority grant aid was often dominated by
a mixture of large grants to long established voluntary organisations such
as Age Concern branches and a patchwork of very small grants to a wide
range of very small voluntary groups. However, local authorities
increasingly had access to time limited grant monies linked to specific
government initiatives. Thus, Chapter Five looked briefly at how joint
finance monies were used to fund a range of new community-based
services. For example, Crossroads Care branches provided practical 'back
up' and relief for informal carers[33]. In the Metropolitan Authority,
Crossroads Care was receiving £23,000 joint finance in 1989/90 towards
the costs of running the project whose aim was:

> ... to recruit and provide care attendants to relieve stress on the family
> or carer of the physically or mentally disabled person and to avoid
> admission to hospital or residential care of the disabled, should support
> arrangements break down[34].

Crossroads Care was also developed in County Council (C) using joint finance monies on the grounds that it was "a vital element in the provision of essential support and relief to family carers"[35].

However, joint finance was not the only source of such monies. Urban authorities with areas of deprivation, such as the London Borough, were able to access urban aid and related grants, some of which were used to fund services for older people. As early as 1975, urban aid was helping to fund a community-based visiting project[36], while in 1981 grants to nine different projects targeted specifically at older people were considered as part of the fourth year of the inner area programme[37]. The main priority chosen was to acquire premises for Age Concern at a cost of £80,000[38]. The Metropolitan Authority was able to fund a welfare rights officer for Age Concern through urban aid monies (interview with General Secretary, Council of Voluntary Service [D], 1973-81).

A third 'special' source of funds related to central government initiatives around such issues as carer support or volunteers. Thus, one of the town/city based Age Concern branches in County Council (B) was initially funded through a Department of Health and Social Security (DHSS) grant relating to volunteers[39], while the Metropolitan Authority was one of the national DHSS pilot projects relating to the coordination of carer support[40]. In terms of the latter, the DHSS grant was used in the following way:

> ... a consortium called ... Caring Together ... was set up by interested people, both professional people and local people, including carers, to actually look at how this money should be allocated and spent. Two development workers were employed to actually do the work and were responsible for reporting back to this consortium. (interview with Director, Voluntary Organisation for Carers [D], 1989-93)

The outcome of this work was the establishment of a new voluntary organisation whose remit was to coordinate carer support within this local authority.

Two key observations need to be made about the use of time-limited grants to fund new mixed economy initiatives in community care. First, it makes such projects very vulnerable at the point when specialist grant monies end. Joint finance agreements seemed to offer stability in terms of the 'pick up' of costs by social services, but this was difficult to enforce in the context of annually renewable/reviewable grants to voluntary organisations. During periods of financial stringency, voluntary organisations were always likely to experience grant cutbacks (interview with Director, Voluntary Organisation for Carers [D], 1989-93). However, one of the clearest examples of a funding crisis in the four case studies was probably the carer coordination scheme in the Metropolitan Authority. The authority was facing a severe financial squeeze and had to work out how to respond to the fact that "during the latter part of 1989, the scheme's funding from time limited resources came to an end and the organisation faced closure". Given that this had been one of the pilot projects in a national DHSS initiative relating to a policy priority area, it was perhaps not surprising that the Social Services Committee decided to approve "a grant of £10,000 for three years (with an annual inflationary increase)"[41]. The carer support scheme survived.

The second key observation is how all four authorities used grants (often initially time limited) to develop what were to become new care services, many of them relating to carer support. Elsewhere in the country, some local authorities were beginning to float off key elements of their in-house domiciliary services such as home care and day care to not for profit agencies. The Metropolitan Authority did this for its residential homes and County Council (B) explored this as a more general strategy, but never progressed it because of a mixture of staff opposition and lack of councillor support (interview with Director of Social Services [B], 1990-93). However, a much less controversial approach was to use the voluntary sector to develop new services, even though they were effectively part of the core community care services of the local authority.

Towards a contract culture?

The emergence of many of these new services run by the voluntary sector coincided with the debate stimulated by the Griffiths Report (1988) and the subsequent White Paper, *Caring for people* (DoH, 1989a) about the need for a contract culture in community care. How did this affect the four case study authorities and their relationship with the voluntary sector?

All four authorities were characterised by taking a strategic view of the rationale for funding voluntary sector organisations, projects and initiatives. In the London Borough, an October 1988 report noted the need for a framework against which to assess the growing volume of grant applications, and indicated that any such framework must recognise both the advocacy role "for the poor and those who are discriminated against" and the fact that government policy and legislation meant "voluntary organisations are increasingly adopting strategic roles in delivering services to the community"[42]. The report concluded that one priority should be to tackle "the scarcity of resources going to organisations for black and ethnic minorities, women, gay men, lesbians and people with disabilities"[43]. Interestingly, the report had earlier analysed grant expenditure for 1988–89 and noted that "projects for and by the elderly are significantly underresourced"[44].

At the corporate level, the London Borough had decided to prioritise advocacy rather than service provision and underrepresented groups rather than traditional client groups. By the late 1980s this was generating tension in the authority with the Director of Social Services informing the Social Services Committee that:

> Community care initiatives are targeted to meet the needs of elderly people, mentally ill people, people with learning difficulties and those needing specialist help such as people who are drug abusers or have AIDS or HIV infection. The point at issue is whether the Council's priorities for grant aid adequately represent the Council's commitment to community care[45].

The report then listed a number of service provider initiatives with the voluntary sector that had not been funded, even when the services had been targeted at underrepresented groups. This suggests a second concern about the need to change the balance between funding for advocacy groups and funding for service provider organisations. The final concern raised in the report was grant length, since most grants were usually only for 12 months:

> The annual grants process is not able to offer sufficiently firm guarantees of ... continuity to projects that provide long-term services. One way of getting around this uncertainty could be to explore ways of setting up core funding on a 'contractual' basis over a fixed period and underpinned by appropriate monitoring and review mechanisms[46].

The Social Services Committee was being asked to begin to consider "more formal partnership arrangements between the statutory and voluntary sectors"[47], with a much increased emphasis on the service provision role of the voluntary sector.

Corporate funding criteria did remain broadly the same, stating that "priority should continue to be given to services provided by and for people who for reasons of race, gender, disability, sexuality and age have been discriminated against or excluded from access to services"[48]. However, social services increasingly interpreted such priorities in terms of service provision rather than advocacy. More specifically, a number of black and minority ethnic community organisations were funded to provide a range of community care services. For example, grants for 1992/93 included luncheon club and meals services for Asian elders and separate day centre provision for Asian elders and for black elders, all run by local community-based organisations[49].

Although it could be argued that this local authority support for such community-based black groups was impressive (interview with Councillor [A], 1964-84), it was certainly not without considerable conflict and dispute. The local authority found itself in repeated arguments with some of the groups in receipt of the largest grants. From the local authority perspective, it was often a simple problem of financial irresponsibility:

> The group has not yet submitted its audited accounts for the year ended 31.3.91. This is a serious breach of the grant aid condition[50].

A different community organisation faced problems of "arrears of tax, NI and rent in the region of £29,000" and was subsequently evicted from its premises[51].

The perspective of workers for these community-based organisations was often very different. A community worker/project manager from that period noted "the usual problems of people just not knowing the system in spite of so many grant officers" (interview with Community Worker/Project Manager [A], 1984-93). As a result, some of the groups were pressed into expanding (for example, from an Asian elders day centre to a full meals on wheels service) before they were ready in terms of the level of accountability expected by the local authority. More specifically, management committee meetings did not happen and there was a "failure to respond in writing to all sorts of things which led to grant cuts and withdrawal and the ultimate collapse of the organisation" (interview with Community Worker/Project Manager [A], 1984-93). Thus, the local authority "may have more equal opportunities jargon than I could ever think of" but the white professionals who work for it "are not even addressing this issue of diversity in any of their processes" (interview with Community Worker/Project Manager [A], 1984-93). Protocols were developed that worked to the advantage of established white organisations like Age Concern and the contract culture served only to further squeeze out small community-based organisations (interview with Community Worker/Project Manager [A], 1984-93).

Pressure to introduce contracts and service agreements rather than grants continued to develop in the early 1990s in the London Borough. Thus, the Social Services Committee was told in April 1992 that "a purchasing strategy for services in the voluntary sector will need to be developed over the next financial year"[52]. The following chapter looks in more detail at how this was developed as part of the process of implementing the community care reforms.

This Committee report also noted that the development of the mixed economy would be helped by the fact that "the voluntary sector is large and very varied" but that "the private sector in social care is still a very small sector of provision"[53]. The authority proved to be very creative with regard to how it might stimulate private sector provision within its boundaries in ways that would be acceptable to those councillors normally very suspicious of this sector. The Director of Social Services explained how the authority would "bend the policies to its own will, so some of the mixed economy staff would find expression in community businesses rather than all out private sector with labels and logos" (interview with Director of Social Services [A], 1986-94). More specifically a proposal was developed as part of the national 'Caring for people who live at home' initiative, the main elements of which were:

- to develop a commercially sound independent community care agency to create and deliver services to black elders and their carers;
- to assist in the development of the black business community;
- to create employment and training opportunities and to maximise the business, financial and professional expertise of local people.

A key expected outcome was the "economic and professional development of an independent social care agency able to compete for commissioned services on an equal footing".

In County Council (B), the growing emphasis on the need for a contract culture led to a review of voluntary sector grants. The Director of Social Services in the late 1980s noted how over £1 million was being spent on annual grants that were normally reviewed each year with an incremental increase, yet his staff "weren't very good at measuring outcomes" and the whole system "was pretty inefficiently managed" (interview with Deputy Director and Director of Social Services [B], 1971-93).

The social services department began making three year grants, but balanced this by insisting that monies were spent on meeting the priorities of the department:

> We tended to try to do it on a rolling basis over a period of three years, or something of that kind, so that at least organisations had knowledge

that they were going to be funded for a period of time, but at the same time they were responding to the sort of directions we felt were most important to them. (interview with Deputy Director and Director of Social Services [B], 1971-93)

However, not all established voluntary organisations were seen as having this capacity to meet departmental priorities and increasingly senior managers were feeling that money "going down that particular hole is not serving any purpose whatever" (interview with Deputy Director and Director of Social Services [B], 1971-93).

Age Concern (B) was seen as coming into this category, especially compared with Age Concern branches in some of the large market towns, which had a clear focus on service provision. Indeed, more generally, an antipathy developed towards county-wide voluntary organisations on the grounds that the local services needed to be commissioned from local voluntary groups by district offices (interview with Deputy Director of Social Services [B], 1989-93). (The next chapter will illustrate how the County believed purchasing and commissioning should occur at a very local level.) "A proper contractual relationship" (interview with Deputy Director of Social Services [B], 1989-93) was established with Age Concern (B) in which only specific services were purchased, which effectively meant a vastly reduced grant. The 1991/92 annual report of Age Concern (B) referred to "our first contractual service", which was a day care initiative in one part of the County[54].

The philosophy of this County was for the private, voluntary and statutory sectors to compete with each other on both quality and price, with the most cost effective winning the most contracts. County Council (B) felt able to operate such a system partly because it had such extensive private residential and nursing home provision. The authority felt it was possible to develop "an open market approach", so long as staff had the ability "to assess the degree of care and/or specialist services required and cost with confidence when seeking to purchase such care"[55]. This was backed up by a system of accreditation based on quality standards for those homes that wished "to contract with the Department for the placement of people who will be financially supported by the Department"[56]. It was to be an approach to the contract culture in which care managers would spot purchase residential and nursing home places for their clients, rather than the local authority contracting a block number of places and then seeking to fill them up (see the next chapter for more details).

County Council (C) and the Metropolitan Authority also recognised the need to move away from the traditional system of annual grants to voluntary organisations. As a report to the Social Services Committee in County Council (C) explained in late 1988:

> Voluntary agencies are major providers of community care for clients in priority groups. At present, their funding is usually from a variety of sources, often temporary or short term, including the Grants Budget. There is a need to identify and secure long term funding for voluntary agencies when short term funding has finished[57].

The approach recommended a few months later was to move to longer-term service agreements where there is "direct service provision provided by voluntary organisations as an alternative to County Council provision"[58].

In a similar vein, the Metropolitan Authority began to take a much more strategic view of its relationships with the voluntary sector in the late 1980s:

> Grants to voluntary organisations in the past have been considered separately to Divisional services, and this has led to both uncertainty and a feeling that voluntary organisations are 'less secure' than the Council's own services. This time grants have had the same scrutiny given to Committee services so that the relationship between the voluntary organisations and the Committee can be seen as a partnership with every organisation's services being considered in the context of that service and not in isolation[59].

More specifically, a system of three year grants was introduced for the major service providers from the voluntary sector (for example, Age Concern, Crossroads Care). Their performance was then reviewed in the third year in terms of aims, staffing, management arrangements, service provision, finance and monitoring. Initial reviews for both Age Concern (D)[60] and Crossroads Care[61] led to a renewal of their grants for three years.

Voluntary organisations as the voice of older people

Not everyone involved in the voluntary sector in the four case studies was delighted by the shift to a contract culture and the emphasis on their service provision role in terms of meeting community care objectives. Some Labour councillors in the London Borough continued to believe that virtually all care services should be provided directly by the local authority (interview with Husband and Wife Labour Councillors [A], 1970-93). The Director of Age Concern (B) complained of how the contract culture squeezed out innovation (interview with Director, Age Concern [B], 1971-93), a view also held by a community worker/project manager involved with small black community organisations in the London Borough (interview with Community Worker/Project Manager [A], 1984-93). The Chief Officer of Age Concern (C1) indicated her relief at leaving her post in 1993 since "social services might be going to become our paymasters and make the running" (interview with Chief Officer, Age Concern [C1], 1981-93). The former General Secretary of the Council of Voluntary Service in the Metropolitan Authority lamented how "care in the community changed forever and a day the whole ethos of the voluntary sector" since "they wanted services out of us" (interview with General Secretary, Council of Voluntary Service [D], 1973-81).

Part of the reason for these doubts was a view that the voluntary sector should provide complementary services to the local authority, rather than core services within a contract culture. However, there was also a view that the voluntary sector had a responsibility to represent the views of older people and sometimes to campaign on their behalf. It is indeed possible to identify such activities from the voluntary sector in all four case studies, but it was an approach that began to sit uncomfortably with the service provider role.

In the London Borough, Age Concern placed considerable emphasis on campaigning on behalf of older people in terms of national issues such as pensions. However, Age Concern (A) also set up a Watchdog Committee on the local authority:

> For instance if there wasn't enough residential care in those days 'why can't we have residential?'... 'What are you doing about home helps? We must have home helps'.... And we pushed and we pushed. (interview with Husband and Wife Labour Councillors [A], 1970-93)

On the whole, it would appear that Labour councillors on the Executive Committee of Age Concern (A) pushed it to be critical of the policies of Conservative governments, especially in so far as they impacted on local services. However, Age Concern (A) also had a high profile in the campaign to reverse cuts in lunch clubs and day centres when the local authority was under Conservative control in the mid-1980s[62].

More generally, it has been seen how the London Borough had a strong commitment to funding advocacy groups, despite the pressure to align grant making to meeting narrowly defined community care objectives. This did encourage the development of a black voluntary sector that was often highly critical of the local authority. In April 1991, a joint seminar was held between this sector and the social services department on the theme of "social services servicing the black community"[63]. The report from this day suggests the recurrence of four main themes/issues:

- accessibility of information about services and function (appropriate language);
- appropriateness of service;
- adequacy of service where there is a disproportionate need amongst black people;
- representation and power of black workers across the council, particularly in policy formulation and decision making[64].

The move to a contract culture was seen by many as likely to squeeze out dissent from the black voluntary sector and to reduce its capacity to be critical of the local authority (interview with Community Worker/Project Manager [A], 1984-93).

County Council (B) saw massive protests over the proposed closure of local authority residential homes (see Chapter Four) and the voluntary sector was very much involved in these campaigns (interview with Chair, Social Services Committee [B], 1989-93). Views on this varied amongst senior social service managers. One commented that one of the greatest concerns of the voluntary sector in the early 1990s was that "if they started taking contracts from us, would they (still) be at the cutting edge of criticism, of challenge, which is a legitimate role for the voluntary sector?" (interview with Director of Social Services [B], 1990-93). Another stressed that the voluntary sector should only be consulted at the district plan level about need and how best to respond to it. However, some voluntary organisations were not happy with this and tried to set up meetings with the Director of Social Services in order to lobby about what was happening at a local level:

> ... they would tend to bring forward sort of complaints that this wasn't happening, that wasn't happening or this change was taking place, will you not do something about it? And of course it took a brave Director to say 'well, if that's the local needs, now that's why it's happening'. (interview with Deputy Director of Social Services [B], 1989-93)

It has been seen earlier in this chapter that the private sector could also be very effective at bringing pressure to bear on the local authority.

The Chief Officer for Age Concern (C1) for most of the study period was quite aware that her organisation had a responsibility to campaign on social care issues that affected the health and welfare of older people. Therefore, at the same time as it was developing a clear service provision role, it was also "very much more involved with actual campaigning on specific issues" (for example, closure of local authority residential homes, increased charges) and "demonstrating outside County Hall" (interview with Chief Officer, Age Concern [C1], 1981-93). The Organising Secretary for Age Concern (C2) also remembered that "there was a terrific number of campaigns" (interview with Organising Secretary, Age Concern [C2], 1971-80).

Such campaigns and demonstrations did cause tensions with the local authority. Age Concern (C1) felt that "we ought to be trying to influence them and on a lot of issues they weren't willing to be influenced and some of the things they were doing we thought really totally wrong" (interview with Chief Officer, Age Concern [C1], 1981-93). Some officers saw this as just part of the emergence of local campaigns that Age Concern (C1) had legitimately decided to join (interview with Joint Commissioner [C], 1992-93). Others were less sanguine. The Director of Social Services noted that "the elderly persons' lobby was quite pronounced" and it "used the media effectively" (interview with Director of Social Services [C], 1988-95) at times of service cuts and residential home closures. However, he remembered how it became necessary "to go through with them the issues around their acting as contractors and not lobbyists and the technical stuff around that".

A number of respondents in the Metropolitan Authority saw a key role of the voluntary sector as being to consult service users and carers (interviews with Health Visitor [D], 1971-93, with Health Visitor [D], 1971-87, and with Director, Voluntary Organisation for Carers [D], 1989-93). It has already been seen how the General Secretary of the Council of Voluntary Service in the 1970s presented this in a challenging way in terms of its implications for statutory agencies through his desire "to bitch like crazy" (interview with General Secretary, Council of Voluntary Service [D], 1973-81). However, the general impression of consultation in the 1980s was of information gathering on behalf of the local authority, rather than in terms of the kind of advocacy and campaigning that characterised some of the other case studies. Indeed, one social services manager was quite explicit that Age Concern (D) had not been a voice for older people because "they've tended to ... be dependent on the local authority, particularly ... for financial support which ... doesn't provide a platform for them to question policy" (interview with Residential and Day Services Officer/District Officer [D], 1985-93).

Conclusion

There has been strong voluntary sector involvement in social care for older people dating back to the 1940s and certainly throughout the 1971–93 study period of this book. As such, there has always been a mixed economy and hence the Conservative governments of the 1980s cannot be given the credit for its establishment. However, the nature of this mixed economy changed significantly in the research period in two main ways. First, the mid-1980s had seen the explosion in private sector residential and nursing home care as a result of the increased availability of social security payments. The second was a movement towards the integration of the voluntary sector into the mainstream of service provision. The emphasis switched from the provision of very general preventative and recreational facilities to service provision for priority groups controlled through contracts and service agreements.

In terms of the four case studies, the London Borough was characterised by the most limited growth of the private sector, while County Council (B) was the most enthusiastic embracer of it. The other two authorities were keen to concentrate on developing the mixed economy through the 'not for profit' sector (including housing associations), rather than the recently established private sector. The London Borough was perhaps the most imaginative in terms of using the voluntary sector to respond to the needs of older people from black and minority ethnic communities. The final section of the chapter suggested that these developments were accompanied by a reduction in the ability of some voluntary organisations to act as a critic of their local authority.

The community care elements of the 1990 NHS and Community Care Act were designed to push this emerging mixed economy into a clear framework underpinned by an emphasis upon markets and competition. How the four case study authorities responded to this challenge is the theme of the next chapter.

Notes

[1] Social Services Committee (A), 26 July 1971 (Section 45, Welfare of the Elderly).

[2] Social Services Committee (B), 30 September 1974 (Position Statement: Social Services).

[3] London Borough (A) (1983) Over 60s Club, *Annual Statement of Accounts.*

[4] Metropolitan Authority (D) (1977) *Volunteers: Policy Report.*

[5] Social Services Committee (D), 22 January 1980 (Policy Statement and Options, 1980-83).

[6] Social Services Committee (D), 18 November 1980 (Luncheon Clubs).

[7] Ibid.

[8] Social Services Department (B), June 1979 (Services for the Elderly in 'B' – A Discussion Document).

[9] Social Services Committee (B), 30 September 1985 (Meals on Wheels Service).

[10] Social Services Committee (B), 19 September 1991 (1991/92 Revenue Budget – Monitoring Report).

[11] Social Services Committee (C), 18 March 1977 (Organised Meals Service).

[12] Ibid.

[13] Social Services Committee (D), 22 January 1980 (Policy Statement and Options, 1980-93).

[14] Social Services Committee (D), 29 March 1976 (WRVS Domiciliary Shopping Service).

[15] Social Services Committee (D), 14 July 1975 (Grants to Voluntary Organisations).

[16] Metropolitan Authority (D) (1974) *The Elderly: A Review of their Needs and Provision for them in the Metropolitan Borough*, September.

[17] Social Services Committee (C), 28 May 1976 (Grants and Subscriptions to Voluntary Organisations).

[18] Social Services Committee (C), 18 March 1977 (Grants and Subscriptions to Voluntary Organisations).

[19] Ibid.

[20] Social Services Committee (C), 27 January 1982 (Age Concern [C1], Annual Report).

[21] Ibid.

[22] Social Services Committee (B), 6 June 1973 (Age Concern).

---

[23] Age Concern (B), *Annual Report, 1991-92*.

[24] Ibid.

[25] Social Services Committee (B), 2 February 1989 (Voluntary Grants Working Party – Age Concern).

[26] Social Services Committee (A), 27 October 1981 (Age Concern Proposals).

[27] Social Services Committee (A), 1 July 1991 (Age Concern Information and Resource Centre and Day Centre for Dementia Sufferers and their Carers).

[28] Social Services Committee (C), 14 June 1971 (Residential Care for the Elderly).

[29] Social Services Committee (C), 5 March 1991 (Elderly Strategy: Replacement Sheltered Housing with Care Scheme).

[30] Social Services Committee (C), 10 December 1991 (Services for Elderly People).

[31] Social Services Committee (A), 19 January 1993 (Commissioning Nursing/ Residential Home Placements).

[32] Social Services Committee (C), 3 March 1992 (Code of Practice for Private Home Care Agencies).

[33] Social Services Committee (D), 27 September 1988 (Review of Grant Aid to Voluntary Organisations).

[34] Ibid.

[35] Social Services Committee (C), 22 November 1988 (Joint Finance – Crossroads Care Attendant Scheme).

[36] Social Services Committee (A), 27 October 1975 (Report of the Urban Aid Grant Sub Committee of Social Services).

[37] Social Services Committee (A), 27 October 1981 (Inner Area Programme: Proposals for Year Four, 1982-83).

[38] Ibid.

[39] Social Services Committee (B), 2 February 1989 (Voluntary Grants Working Party: Age Concern).

[40] Social Services Committee (D), 2 August 1988 (Caring Together).

[41] Social Services Committee (D), 17 September 1991 (Carer Support Scheme).

[42] Social Services Committee (A), 31 October 1988 (Grants Strategy, 1989-90).

[43] Ibid.

[44] Ibid.

[45] Social Services Committee (A), 31 January 1989 (Main Programme Grant Aid 1989/90 to Voluntary Organisations).

[46] Ibid.

[47] Ibid.

[48] Social Services Committee (A), 11 February 1992 (Grants to Voluntary Organisations).

[49] Ibid.

[50] Ibid.

[51] Ibid.

[52] Social Services Committee (A), 27 April 1992 (Social Services Department – Service Plan, 1992-93).

[53] Ibid.

[54] Age Concern (B), *Annual Report, 1991-92.*

[55] Social Services Committee (B), 19 September 1991 (Elderly Services Development Programme).

[56] Social Services Committee (B), 18 June 1992 (Contracting for Residential and Nursing Home Care).

[57] Social Services Committee (C), 22 November 1988 (Joint Finance Strategy).

[58] Social Services Committee (C), 8 March 1989 (Financial Support to Voluntary Organisations).

[59] Social Services Committee (D), 21 March 1989 (Service Charges in 1989/90).

[60] Social Services Committee (D), 23 July 1991 (Age Concern 'D').

[61] Social Services Committee (D), 28 May 1991 (Crossroads Care Attendant Scheme).

[62] *Lunch Clubs Axed – Social Services Cuts Continue,* Newspaper of Age Concern (A), October 1985.

[63] Social Services Committee (A), 8 April 1991 (Social Services Serving the Black Community).

[64] Ibid.

SEVEN

Towards quasi-markets in community care

Introduction

The last chapter looked at the development of the mixed economy of social care in the four case studies. This chapter takes the analysis one stage further by looking at how the four authorities responded to the change agenda required by the 1990 NHS and Community Care Act. More specifically it will look at their approach to establishing what Le Grand and others have called quasi-markets (Bartlett et al, 1994; Le Grand and Bartlett, 1993).

What are quasi-markets?

The previous chapter looked at the growth of the voluntary and private sectors as key providers of social care services within a contract or service agreement culture. These types of development were strongly supported by both the Griffiths Report (1988) and the subsequent White Paper, *Caring for people* (DoH, 1989a). Both had argued that the contract culture needed to occur in the context of social services authorities being given the lead agency role for a wide range of groups including older people. However, the lead agency role was not about the monopoly provision of services but rather the further development of a mixed economy of social care based largely on the independent sector. As already indicated, many commentators at the time saw this declining emphasis on the state as service provider as part of a long-term strategy to privatise welfare (Biggs, 1990/91; Langan, 1990).

The publications by Le Grand and his colleagues in the early 1990s had referred to such developments as quasi rather than pure markets, and pointed out that they were also being introduced into other areas of the welfare state such as education and the health service. But what are quasi-markets? Propper et al (1994) argued that the main quasi-market reforms of the early 1990s had a number of common features:

- the separation of purchaser and provider functions within each service;
- the devolution of managerial autonomy to individual provider units;
- changes to funding mechanisms based either on the introduction of formula funding or a system of contracting between purchasers and providers.

The approach taken by the Conservative government to welfare reform implementation stressed that efficiency, effectiveness and responsiveness would flow from increased competition within a market. However, the community care and other welfare reforms of the period created quasi rather than pure markets since:

> In contrast to standard markets, these systems remain free at the point of delivery: no money changes hands between the final user (eg pupils, patients) and the provider of services (eg schools, hospitals). Thus the state has retained its role as a funder of services within the welfare state, but the task of providing has been transferred from an integrated set of state owned and managed enterprises to a variety of independent provider organisations including not for profit organisations, private companies and state owned units under devolved management. (Propper et al, 1994, pp 1-2)

Although this comment can be challenged on the grounds that fees are charged for many social care services (domiciliary ones as well as residential/nursing care), it still indicates how the community care reforms were based on a belief in markets and competition, even though they did not usher in full privatisation. The system remained heavily funded and heavily subsidised by the state. In many cases, the fees charged were no reflection of real costs.

Implementing quasi-markets in community care: an overview

The community care reforms outlined in the White Paper (DoH, 1989a) and confirmed by the 1990 Act were far reaching and complex. Not only was there a general shift to a mixed economy of providers, but there was also a very specific requirement on local authorities to take over the funding of independent sector residential and nursing home care from the social security system (see Chapter One). The main policy guidance became available in 1990 and covered such diverse implementation issues as community care planning, care management and assessment, and commissioning and purchasing (DoH, 1990).

The main response of government to the concerns of local authorities about the implications of this challenging agenda was to phase in implementation so that the production of community care plans on an annual basis did not become a requirement until April 1992 and the social security changes did not take effect until April 1993. Earmarked monies were also set aside by the government to meet the costs of (i) the new residential and nursing home responsibilities and (ii) the general costs of developing a new community care infrastructure. However, many authorities were not convinced that such monies were adequate and were suspicious about how long they would remain earmarked. Thus, the Metropolitan Authority was worried that although they were to get £2.12 million in 1993/94:

> The allocation for 1994-5 has not yet been announced. Committee have already been advised that the evidence suggests there are major causes for concern about the amount of the transfer for 1994-5 and for 1995-6, the final year of the ring fencing of the transferred funding[1].

It should be remembered that the community care reforms were being implemented during a period of considerable financial stringency for local authorities. Social services felt they were being asked to develop a new approach to community care at a time when their core budgets were being cut.

Financial worries also existed for the other three local authorities. For example, County Council (B) expressed general concern as early as June 1988 about the "increasing signs that sources of funds for existing programmes of community care are becoming more inaccessible"[2]. The Social Services Committee of County Council (C) was discussing major cutbacks to the overall budget at the same time as planning its community care reform implementation strategy. The Director of Social Services remembers "cutting budgets under great financial restraint" (interview with Director of Social Services [C], 1988-95) and hence it was necessary to tell members:

> ... that they spend their budget in a few limited blocks of expenditure such as Elderly Persons' Homes.... Achievement of this Committee's budget targets is therefore inevitably going to involve reductions in those large blocks of expenditure; Committee will be only too aware

that cuts in virtually all of these blocks ... would be very unpopular and have a severe impact on elderly and disabled people in the county[3].

The London Borough not only faced significant cutback pressures of its own but was also worried about how difficult it was to predict the financial implications of the new system, partly because this would depend on decisions by NHS trusts with regard to the future provision of continuing care beds[4] (see also Chapter Five).

Research by Wistow et al (1992) showed that local authorities varied in their attitudes and enthusiasm for the reforms. They identified 10 different models of provision of community care (see Figure 7.1) and found enormous variation in attitudes to the reforms and their organisational implications:

> While it would be wrong to generalise too freely, there were some clear and largely predictable rankings in attitudes towards these options. Thus most Labour authorities preferred d to e, and strongly preferred e to f. Indeed, option f was a non-starter in some authorities. If the possibility was mentioned, they also ruled out j and were often unhappy about it. To take another example, most Conservative authorities supported option g, expressed some practical but not ideological reservations about h, and usually liked the idea of e and f in principle even though elected members had some difficulty supporting the sale of facilities in their own wards. Option c hardly ever received support from either officers or members, and it was too early for local authorities to make any judgements about the viability of option j. These are gross generalisations, and only rarely were two authorities alike. Indeed, one of the strong conclusions to emerge from our study was that generalisations along party political lines are often hard to sustain. (Wistow et al, 1992, p 30)

The four case study authorities in this research reflected something of this diversity, although all of them shared concerns about the future of in-house services. Most Labour councillors in the London Borough remained very suspicious of the mixed economy thrust of the reforms because of their implications for the traditional service delivery role of the local authority. The Director of Social Services remembered an attitude of "we must promote in house services" (interview with Director of Social Services [A], 1986-94), while the Director of Age Concern in that authority in the early 1990s felt that her organisation was pushing the

Figure 7.1: A simple catalogue of potential alternative modes of provision of community care

a. Continuing local authority provision as it is currently organised, with no planned changes to the management, funding or regulation of activities.

b. Continuing local authority provision with reorganisation of the Social Services Department (SSD) along the lines of a purchaser/provider split of some kind and to some degree.

c. Management or staff buy-outs of some local authority services.

d. Floating off some services to a not for profit trust which allows the local authority to retain some degree of control, though with eligibility for Department of Social Security (DSS) payments.

e. Selling off services, perhaps at a nominal price, to voluntary organisations (new or already working in the authority), which act independently of the authority, except for any service agreements or contracts.

f. Selling off services to private (for profit) agencies (new or already with a presence in the authority), which act independently of the authority, except for any service agreements or contracts.

g. Encouraging (or perhaps simply not stopping) voluntary or not for profit organisations setting up new services.

h. Encouraging (or perhaps simply not stopping) private (for profit) agencies setting up new services.

i. Considering Health Authorities as potential providers for some social care services, such as residential care for older people or people with mental health problems.

j. Bringing NHS trusts into the supply picture.

Source: Based on Wistow et al (1992, p 30)

mixed economy much more than the local authority (interview with Director, Age Concern [A], 1990-93) (see also Chapter Six).

County Council (B) tended to take a positive attitude from the outset towards community care reform. Its 1986 reorganisation into 32 districts was seen by most senior managers as very much in keeping with the philosophy of the Griffiths Report (1988) and the community care White Paper (DoH, 1989a). This reorganisation had been based on two principles:

> One was to decentralise so that the organisation at local level was able to understand local needs and be able to respond to them locally.... And the second was that there should be an integration of services so as to be able to respond to those needs more flexibly. (interview with Deputy Director of Social Services [B], 1989-93)

This authority was already beginning to explore care management approaches before the publication of the Griffiths Report. Where there was less agreement in this authority was on how far to push the quasi-market element of the mixed economy. More specifically, how much protection should in-house services receive in the face of competition from independent providers?

The 1986 restructuring in County Council (B) was partly driven by a belief that people were allocated the services available rather than what they required. Community care was service rather than user driven. This view was also widely held in County Council (C) where one senior manager remarked how "we were very much in sympathy with all the Griffiths reforms" because social workers, home help organisers, meals on wheels organisers and district nurses were assessing people for a specific service or services rather than "looking at ... needs as a whole" (interview with Principal Officer (Elderly Services), Social Services [C], 1989-93). The Director of Social Services for that period took a more cynical view. The community care reforms may have been theoretically right, but "in reality it was all about public expenditure control" (interview with Director of Social Services [C], 1988-95) in terms of the social security budget.

The Metropolitan Authority was like County Council (B) in seeing its move to a more decentralised approach as very much in keeping with the philosophy of the community care reforms:

> Three years ago, [the] Social Services Division established six geographical area teams responsible for the majority of services to their local communities. This was a deliberate move to make services more accessible, more local and more responsive to the needs of the local communities[5].

A new Director of Social Services in 1987 had been brought in with a remit to see "decision making devolved to the areas" and this had included "getting rid of the residential and fieldwork divide which had been very strong" (interview with Director of Social Services [D], 1987-93). However, this was also an authority very proud of its in-house services and so members were very protective of these services in a similar way to councillors from the London Borough.

The rest of this chapter looks at specific aspects of reform implementation, namely development of purchaser and provider splits, contracting with the independent residential and nursing home sector, and broad approaches to assessment and care management. It will be seen that much of the planning for April 1993 was very rushed and compressed into the autumn of 1992 and the spring of 1993. As the Metropolitan Authority noted, most social services departments had "only started serious work in preparation for implementation in the autumn ...

because of a substantial delay caused by election fever"[6]. This was supported in another study by one of the authors of this book in which senior managers from social services and other key agencies had stressed that "the likelihood of a General Election made strategic long term thinking difficult and unattractive" (Hoyes et al, 1992, p 58).

In some authorities, such election fever enabled those hostile to the reforms to block proposals from senior staff to implement radical care management or purchaser–provider split change. But it also generated caution in others because of the possibility of a major policy reversal in the event of an election of a Labour government in 1992. This, of course, did not happen. Instead, the Conservatives were returned, which resulted in the Department of Health speeding up the availability of policy and practice guidance to local authorities. This led one of the four case studies to complain about the "enormous amount of official and semi-official guidance which has been received" that was only serving to create "some confusion"[7]. One reason for confusion was that much of the guidance received on contracting, care management and the rest was just that, namely guidance rather than instruction. Local authorities were left with enormous discretion about how they reorganised their own departments and their relationships with others. Three key aspects of this turbulent situation are outlined in this chapter.

Towards a purchaser–provider split?

As indicated above, quasi-markets are based on a belief in the cost effectiveness of getting a number of providers to compete for business from a single purchaser, namely the social services department. It has already been seen how the private residential and nursing home sector tended to be suspicious of local authorities as favouring their own residential homes and that some local authorities were indeed concerned to protect their 'in-house' provision.

From the outset, the government flagged up its concern about this issue. The White Paper on community care decided against an extension of compulsory competitive tendering to local authority social care services, but instead favoured a greater use of service specifications, agency agreements and contracts in an evolutionary way. It went on to argue that this was "likely to require a clear distinction to be made between the purchasing and providing functions within a local authority" (DoH, 1989a, p 23).

The policy guidance of the following year took this one stage further by making clear that:

> In potential terms in developing the enabling role authorities will need to distinguish between aspects of work in SSDs concerned with
>
> • the assessment of individuals' needs, the arrangement and purchase of services to meet them
>
> and
>
> • direct service provision. It will be important that this distinction is reflected within the SSD's management structure at both the 'macro' level (involving plans to meet strategic priorities as a whole) and at the 'micro' level (where services are being arranged for individuals). (DoH, 1990, pp 37-8)

In other words, all local authorities were expected to demonstrate how they were splitting their purchasing and providing functions.

To help them in the process, the government commissioned a private management consultancy firm to look at options and this led to a specification and elaboration of a number of models rather than a requirement to follow any specific mould (Price Waterhouse/DoH, 1991). More specifically, three broad approaches to establishing a split were outlined:

• strategic purchaser/commissioner and provider separation;
• purchaser/commissioner and provider separation at senior management team level;
• localised purchaser/commissioner and provider separation.

These three approaches are illustrated in Figure 7.2, and it will be seen how the four case studies reflected something of this diversity in their own attempts to establish purchaser–provider splits.

As already indicated, the London Borough initially took a cautious view of the reforms because of the central concern of members to protect what they considered to be excellent local authority in-house services (interview with Director of Social Services [A], 1986-94). This ensured considerable hostility to any idea of a purchaser–provider split and so proposals were made for restructuring with a rather different emphasis. As the Director of Social Services at the time explained:

> Well I seem to remember ... drawing up a structure which wasn't a
> conventional purchaser/provider split but had commissioning and
> inspection within it and quality assurance.... So it was a slight attempt
> at putting providers in a separate organisational arrangement but it
> certainly wasn't an internal market in the way that some authorities
> went for broke. (interview with Director of Social Services [A], 1986–
> 94)

As a result, members were open to persuasion that quality assurance meant
that in-house services needed to meet the same standards as the
independent sector, even if they were not required to go through the
same contracting process (interview with Director of Social Services [A],
1986–94).

Initial proposals for restructuring went before the Social Services
Committee in July 1991. This included the new Division of Quality
Assurance and Planning to include the inspection and registration function,
the race unit, strategic planning, community care planning and a new
function of service commissioning. With regard to the latter, members
were told that:

> The new 'commissioning unit' would assume the role of managing the
> contracts with the department's residential care when transferred, service
> level agreements where they exist with the voluntary sector, compulsory
> competitive tendering contracts and any other commissioning of service
> which might take place in the future[8].

The commissioning role was further clarified in October 1992 when it
was made clear that the commissioning role included "working towards
a contract/service level agreement approach in commissioning the
Department's own directly managed services"[9]. Another task was to
encourage the development of new and different services from both the
private and voluntary sectors that would be based on service level
agreements. This emphasis on the achievement of quality through service
specifications was further emphasised with the formal establishment of a
quality standards section within the Quality Assurance and Planning
Division[10].

Research by Lewis and Glennerster (1996) in the same authority
suggested that both the Director of Social Services and the Assistant
Director who headed the Division saw commissioning as having the
capacity to enhance equal opportunities "and to stimulate new provision
for those whose experience of traditional services had been negative,

Figure 7.2: Possible departmental structures under the three approaches

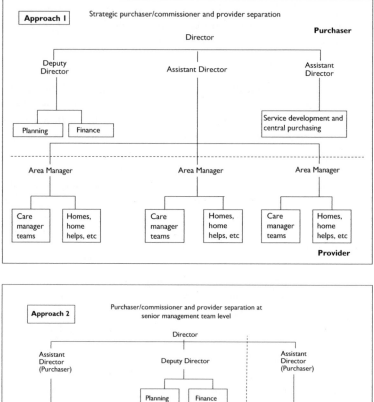

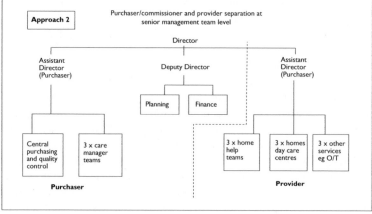

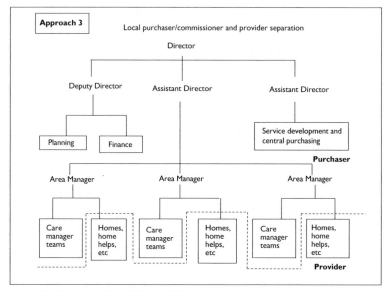

Source: Price Waterhouse/DoH (1991, pp 32-3)

particularly black and minority users" (p 58). Despite sensitivities around the need to protect in-house services, Lewis and Glennerster (1996) stress the bullish tone of the new Division because of its emphasis on securing the best service irrespective of the supplier.

It has already been seen how County Council (B) had been involved in a radical decentralisation of its services during the 1980s. It was, therefore, perhaps no surprise when it decided to create a purchaser–provider split of all functions, including childcare, at the level of its 32 district offices[11]. During 1990-91, three pilot programmes were established prior to what was expected to be a phased county-wide reorganisation over a three year period (Hoyes et al, 1994). At its simplest, care management teams became the purchasers of services on behalf of clients from either in-house provider teams, which were district based, or from the independent sector. The central importance of the care management teams was to be emphasised through the delegation of budgetary control. District managers were expected to play a pivotal role by coordinating information on local need and "by using contracts with service providers to ensure that services develop in response"[12]. One of the aims of the three pilot programmes was to explore different ways in which this might best be achieved.

By April 1993, it seemed that these changes were to be pushed further forward:

> ... the county was planning further structural changes to consolidate
> and strengthen the purchasing function, and to develop and support
> the management structure of the in-house providers. The main effect
> of this restructuring would be a reduction in the number of districts
> from 32 to 19, and the establishment of a managerially separate provider
> division, known as 'Community Services – County Council B'[13].

Despite this long-standing commitment to radical change, the implementation of a purchaser–provider split proved to be highly controversial.

The Deputy Director of Social Services remembered how "for 18 months we sort of messed around arguing between ourselves about this" (interview with Deputy Director of Social Services [B], 1989-93). Initial disagreements had been about whether or not the district manager could manage both the purchasing and providing arms of their district. This respondent believed that the key role of such individuals was to manage purchasing in the interests of the service user and within overall resource constraints. There was a danger of this being compromised if this role also covered service provision, and in any case "economies of scale are such in lots of services you couldn't do it at a District level" (interview with Deputy Director of Social Services [B], 1989-93). This view eventually prevailed so that "the County Council's own services [were] ... put together in one lump" (interview with Deputy Director of Social Services [B], 1989-93).

Nevertheless, the eventual purchaser–provider split chosen was still a radical one, as shown by Figure 7.3. The new structure made a clear distinction between purchasing and commissioning tasks and those associated with in-house provision. It also needs to be noted how this new structure confirmed that the purchaser–provider split should include childcare as well as adult services.

County Council (B) faced another controversial issue with regard to the purchaser–provider split as a result of its belief in the virtues of competition between providers in (quasi) markets. It had to decide on the nature of the competition between in-house services and the independent sector. The London Borough had restricted itself to stressing that in-house services needed to meet the same quality service specifications as other providers, but used the independent (and mainly the voluntary) sector to develop new services. County Council (B) was tempted to go much further and force in-house services to compete for social care business on the basis of price as well as quality, and through contracts that gave no long-term guarantee of business. Private residential

Figure 7.3: Proposed management structure for County Council (B) (from 1 April 1993)[14]

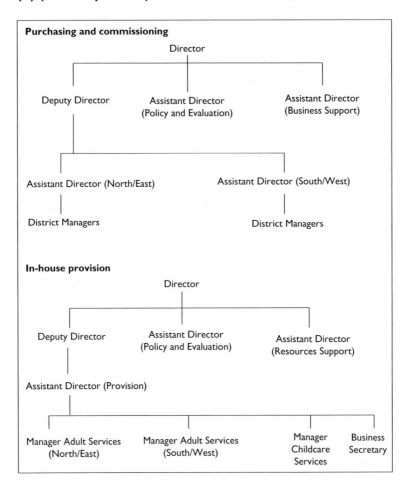

and nursing homes were particularly aggressive in complaining about unfair competition from local authority services (interview with Director of Social Services [B], 1990-93). Full competition was never imposed, despite a Conservative majority on the Council during much of this period. However, subsequent "changes to conditions of employment of staff" were pushed through by the following Liberal Democrat Council in order "to make them a bit more competitive" (interview with Deputy Director of Social Services [B], 1989-93). Nevertheless, the end result was much closer to the position of the London Borough than one might have expected. The County may have espoused a "business excellence model" (interview with Director of Social Services [B], 1990-93). However, it was one based on agreed quality standards for all provider sectors, rather than one in which in-house services risked going out of business if they lacked price competitiveness. Indeed, by November 1992, it had produced a Quality Standard Directory, which covered everything from care management to nursing home provision from a belief "that everyone – the user, manager, worker, councillor and man or woman in the street [should] know what we mean by quality and the nature of service standards"[15].

County Council (C) decided to carry out a major restructuring of its social services but one that was quite cautious in terms of the establishment of a purchaser–provider split at the field level. In autumn 1992, its five geographical divisions were reduced to three and a central commissioning unit was created, led by a new post of Assistant Director (Commissioning and Planning). This clear split between purchasing and providing functions at the macro level was not fully mirrored at the divisional level. As Hoyes et al (1994) explain:

> Within each of the three divisions, new care manager teams for adults were formed.... However, most team members retain a mixture of purchaser and provider functions. (p 9)

Having said this, a clear purchaser–provider split was established with regard to the home care service through "a reshaping to separate care management and service management within the overall domiciliary service"[16]. However, this was for pragmatic as much as ideological reasons – there was a pressing need "to allow for care management resources to be released"[17] through the re-designation of some home care organisers as care managers. More specifically 14 home care organiser posts and 22 assistant home care organiser posts were to be reduced to 14 domiciliary care manager posts to manage the provider teams and 22 care manager posts to focus on assessment and purchasing.

Within the authority there was considerable concern about the need to protect high quality in-house provision. For this reason it was decided not to allow individual care managers to be budget holders nor to set up provider units as separate trading accounts, even though there was an aspiration to move in that direction in the future.

In terms of contracting, this meant that for some there was an illusion of radical change in the 1992/93 period. A senior manager remembered how:

> We had this classic anecdote of burning out all the photocopiers because we had to move overnight from no purchasing to contracting with 200 providers and we'd never done this before, so we had to make up all the mechanisms and all the contracts and send them out ready. (interview with Principal Officer (Elderly), Social Services [C], 1989-93)

The reality was that it was "a damp squib with 1ˢᵗ April ... just the same as 31ˢᵗ March" (interview with Principal Officer (Elderly), Social Services [C], 1989-93). This respondent felt that the really significant moves to a purchaser–provider split occurred later in the mid-1990s, although some of this was prefigured in the study period through early discussions about approaches to joint commissioning with health[18].

The Metropolitan Authority had been through an extensive restructuring of its social services in the late 1980s. This took the same approach as County Council (B), in that decision making was devolved to area offices and the new structure removed the residential and fieldwork divide which had been very strong (interview with Director of Social Services [D], 1987-93).

However, the new structure was not based on a clear division between purchasing and provider functions and this led to pressure for further change. As the Director of Social Services explained to his committee:

> Over recent months the District Auditors have been piloting a new audit on preparation for Community Care, and (this authority) has been one of the authorities in which they have undertaken their pilot study. The draft report was critical of the proposals for the structure of Adult Services in the Division, and recommended that consideration be given to the separation of the purchaser and provider functions at a higher level of management[19].

The proposed new structure is outlined in Figure 7.4. It was argued that the benefits of this new structure would include:

- a greater emphasis on the distinction of roles between purchasing and providing;
- less conflict for service managers when developing new services;
- the pairing of development roles between purchaser and provider;
- coterminosity and consistency with children's services[20].

From community care to market care?

Figure 7.4: Adult services structure (Metropolitan Authority)[21]

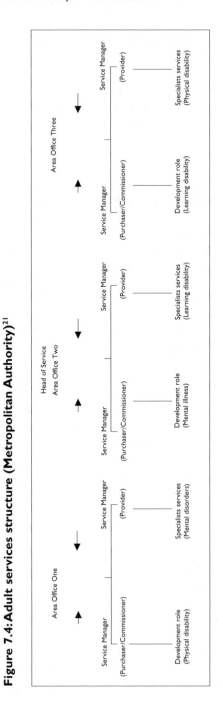

However, it took some considerable time for these changes to be finally agreed and introduced. A working group was established to explore "the implications for the organisation, structure and management of the Division of applying the clarification of rules of Purchasers and Commissioners from Providers"[22]. The eventual reorganisation took place over a three month period in spring 1992 and it was hoped that the new structure would "be a major initiative in clarifying the rules and functions of assessment as distinct from the provision of services"[23].

Contracting with the independent residential and nursing home sector

Chapter Four looked in detail at the changing role of local authority residential care but set this in the context of the rapid growth of independent sector provision from the mid-1980s onwards. As has been shown earlier, a key feature of the *Caring for people* White Paper on community care (DoH, 1989a) and the subsequent 1990 Act was the introduction of a new funding regime for people seeking public support to enter private and voluntary sector nursing and residential homes. This was to become the responsibility of local authorities and funded through a transfer of money from the social security budget to local authorities. However, the hope was that local authorities would have discretion to use some of this money to establish 'at home' care packages and hence reduce the numbers going into institutional care. Local authorities were offered support in this role through the issuing of guidance on the purchase of services, which covered issues such as developing service specifications and writing and monitoring contracts (DoH, 1991).

The sums of money transferred to local authorities were considerable, as can be seen from Table 7.1. These figures were not announced until autumn 1992 (DoH, 1992), the lateness partly reflecting the fierceness of

Table 7.1: Social security transfer money to local authorities (1993-96)

	Cumulative amount (£ million)	Annual amount (£ million)
1993-94	399	399
1994-95	1,050	651
1995-96	1,568	518

Note: Figures rounded to the nearest million.
Source: DoH (1992)

the debate about the principles which should underpin the share of this money allocated to individual local authorities. Should these allocations be driven by estimates of the need of local populations for such care or existing patterns of provision by the independent sector? The chosen approach was complex. The government decided that 50% of the social security transfer money should be allocated according to existing Department of Social Security expenditure on institutional care. The remaining 50% would be needs based through a standard spending assessment (SSA) formula. The memorandum announcing this explained that the new system would not "threaten the viability of both existing and future care arrangements of residents in homes" (DoH, 1992, p 5). However, in due course the social security transfer monies were to be 100% integrated into the SSA formula, so that the short-term 'protection' of existing institutional care would be combined with the long-term objective of shifting patterns of provision to better reflect patterns of need. Finally, the memorandum indicated that 75% of the overall grant to each local authority (both the social security transfer money and more general transitional cost monies) should be spent on paying for care provided by the independent sector. This could be either institutional care or domiciliary services.

The reference to a needs led versus a provision led allocation of social security monies to local authorities is, of course, illusory. The whole point of the reforms was that expenditure on residential and nursing home care under the 1990 Act was to be ring-fenced, unlike the old social security system. However, this could create problems for those authorities with very small independent sector provision (the London Borough) and those with extensive provision (County Council B). This had far-reaching implications for the London Borough whose very small financial allocation reflected its tiny number of registered home places. The authority felt it had simply been allocated too little money and this made it very difficult to implement the new funding regime given the overall financial problems of the local authority. Table 7.2 sets out the large estimated shortfalls in the first two years, which were seen as "the cause of considerable concern"[24].

At first glance, County Council (B) was in a more favourable position than the London Borough since its social security transfer allocation was considerable given the large number of registered places. However, this has to be set against the size of the sector in this County and the fact that over time it was aware that the formula for allocation would shift to one based on need, rather than one based on the historical legacy of an enormous 'inherited' independent sector provision. The local authority

Table 7.2: Shortfall in residential and nursing home monies (London Borough)[25]

| | Annual total cost | | | | | |
| | 1993/94 | | 1994/95 | | 1995/96 | |
	FTE nos	Cost	FTE nos	Cost	FTE nos	Cost
Nursing homes	120	£1.13m	264	£2.53m	217	£3.64m
Residential care	192	£1.65m	423	£3.70m	507	£4.36m
Other adults – transferred cases	30	£0.04m	37	£0.05m	45	£0.06m
Costs of 'waiting lists'	4	£0.01m	8	£0.02m	8	£0.02m
Cost of alignment of charges		£0.03m		£0.04m		£0.06m
Totals		£3.33m		£6.97m		£8.08m
Estimated transfer		£1.02m		£4.08m		£9.00m
Shortfall		£2.13m		£2.17m		(£0.02m)

Note: These figures do not appear to add up, but are an accurate reflection of the report to the Social Services Committee.

had the challenge of managing a reduction in public expenditure in this sector, which was bound to lead to a contraction and the closure of some homes. The chair of the Social Services Committee remembered there being "47 private homes in (town X) and they were all struggling" (interview with Chair, Social Services Committee [B], 1989-93).

The Director of Social Services noted how:

> Once it transferred to community care legislation, we knew for the first time it was cash limited.... What the Government wanted us to do ... was to stop the spiral of expenditure. So in [County Council B] you had a growing residential market, a huge market which was still growing. With a reduced budget, there was bound to be a squeeze. (interview with Director of Social Services [B], 1990-93)

Returning to the position of the London Borough, it may have been concerned about the shortfall it faced, but it was clear that it had no alternative but to accept that the government required it to use a range of in-house and independent sector provision. This was because of the requirement that 75% of the earmarked community care grant to individual local authorities had to be spent on the independent sector.

As explained in the previous chapter, the authority, therefore, recognised that it needed to commission places in the independent sector from outside the borough, and it decided to do this by commissioning 40% of its beds on a block basis from those homes most regularly used by local residents[26]. The remaining 60% of nursing and residential home places and all the adult places were to be 'spot purchased' on an individual basis from an approved list of 150 independent sector homes.

The 10 homes in the preferential block purchase position were chosen through a mapping exercise, which identified them as within the maximum affordable fee range of the local authority, and were also seen by users, carers and professionals as providing quality care. Two of these homes were also selected "because of their sensitivity in meeting the placement needs of black residents"[27].

A feature of the London Borough approach was to emphasise the importance of quality standards to be monitored by the newly created Quality Assurance and Planning Division (see discussion above). This meant approved residential and nursing homes had to demonstrate that they met quality standards in such areas as:

- complaints procedure;
- equality of opportunity recruitment policy;
- systems for addressing racism and sexism;
- choice for the resident.

County Council (B) also wished to place great emphasis on quality service standards for residential care[28] and was able to do so in the knowledge that it was in a strong position to insist upon such standards. The County had a surplus of residential and nursing home places. Most homes would be desperate to have places purchased by the local authority. The strategy was to create a high threshold of quality before a home could be approved. Those approved could have their beds purchased on a 'spot' basis by individual care managers on behalf of their clients.

The proposed standards covered a wide range of areas, including:

- a personal contract and care plan with which individuals agree to ensure that individual needs are met;
- the opportunity to review care arrangements with the care manager and the manager of the home at least annually;
- a home based on good foundations such as clear written policies on aims and objectives;

- quality guarantees in daily living such as "personal choice in all aspects of individual lifestyle, ample opportunity for self expression and assistance to make informed choices and decisions"[29];
- built in safeguards such as the right to see records maintained on the individual's behalf.

The standards were the outcome of extensive consultation including the private sector (interview with Chair, Private Residential Care Homes Association [B], 1985-93) and led to the establishment of a formal accreditation system by the County. This was seen as essential by social services since:

> ... how would you give advice to an elderly person in hospital if our staff had never been into a private home? What you then have to have is a system because you can't leave it to the individual to decide whether they 'like' the home or not, so to be fair to the home owner, it had to be on an agreed system. (interview with Director of Social Services [B], 1990-93)

The Director of Social Services for that period had hoped for a more elaborate accreditation system that gave stars according to the quality of provision, but this became squeezed out "through the mill of negotiation with the hundreds of associations" (interview with Director of Social Services [B], 1990-93). The chosen system of accreditation instead used the Quality Standards Directory approach to encourage the service user, carer and care manager to ask penetrating questions about the quality of care available in homes under consideration.

In County Council (C), there was "not a lot of involvement with the private sector pre 93" and so relations with social services just "tinkered along" (interview with Director of Social Services [C], 1988-95). However, the task of establishing a communications system was considerable. Nursing home proprietors were formed into a county-wide association, but independent sector residential homes (and the 16 home care agencies) had to be contacted on a one-to-one basis[30]. One consequence of this was that it was quite late before any clear decisions were made on the new contracting arrangements. In September 1992, the Social Services Committee was being informed that on the basis of the work of the commissioning unit, it would be possible "to advise the Committee in December on the extent of contracting, the methods of contracting, and the likely process that will need to be adopted"[31]. However, the December meeting was merely told that "detailed discussions and negotiations [with the independent sector] will continue over the winter"[32]. It proved very difficult for the private sector providers to agree a common price basis for negotiation with the County, so the latter in the end imposed a price, having checked with other local authorities that it was not way out of line (interview with Director of Social Services [C], 1988-95).

In the Metropolitan Authority, regular meetings were "held with owners of private residential care homes and nursing homes and a dialogue [was] maintained about the authority's approach to purchasing care from 1st April"[33]. More specifically discussions focused around agreeing a contract for care, specifying standards and agreeing a new fee structure. However, maintaining a dialogue was to prove difficult with a "very high level of anxiety within the independent sector" because of the need "to consider how best to address a planned reduction of the overall level of provision of residential care and nursing home care"[34] in the authority. The aspiration was to establish an approved list of homes working to an enhanced specification.

Despite these tensions it proved possible for the local authority to agree a maximum price for each level of care "that is within estimated costs and that enables [the local authority] to purchase care from the majority of homes without the necessity of any 'top up' payments by a relative or carer"[35].

Agreeing a contract price was an important issue for this authority because of the creation of a 'not for profit' body to run its former local authority residential homes. A block contract was held with this organisation to purchase all its beds. The local authority needed to demonstrate a common price for all the residential care to the rest of the independent residential home sector, even though beds in the rest of the sector were only being bought on a spot purchase rather than a block contract basis. In the first six weeks of the new arrangements, social services "made contractual arrangements to purchase care for over 70 people in the independent sector"[36].

Assessment, care management and eligibility for services

The rationale behind the introduction of the purchaser–provider split into social services departments was partly that they needed to be seen to be dealing with the independent sector in an even-handed way compared to the local authority when considering the purchase of services on behalf of clients. Closely linked to this was the emphasis on user assessment and the need to purchase only those services that the client really wanted and at the minimum available price. The final section of this chapter illustrates how the authorities in the four case study areas attempted to achieve this and how their efforts were complicated by the need to ensure that user-led assessment did not result in a major overspend on the community care budget. User-centred assessment and care management were seen as needing to be balanced against the strict application of eligibility criteria.

As already indicated, social services departments were not short of guidance about how they might go about tackling these tasks. For example, the Department of Health produced guides for both practitioners (DoH/Social Services Inspectorate, 1991b) and managers (DoH/Social Services Inspectorate, 1991a) on care management and assessment. Both guides defined care management as "the process of tailoring services to individual needs" (DoH/Social Services Inspectorate, 1991a, p 11) within which assessment was only one of seven different stages (see Figure 7.5).

Figure 7.5: The process of care management

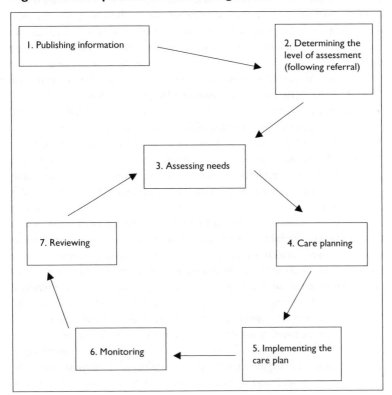

Source: DoH/SSI (1991a, p 12)

The guides re-emphasised that care management began with needs rather than with services, with need being defined as:

> ... the requirements of individuals to enable them to achieve, maintain or restore an acceptable level of social independence or quality of life, as defined by the particular care agency or authority. (p 14)

But need was also defined as a dynamic concept that would vary over time according not only to changes in national legislation, changes in local policy and patterns of local demand, but also in terms of "the availability of resources" (p 14). As a result needs should "be explicitly defined and prioritised in policy statements" and elected members had "to ensure on a continuing basis that they are able to resource the response to the needs for which they accept any responsibility" (p 14).

How did the four case study authorities respond? The London Borough put great emphasis on pilot care management schemes[37] with a view that the best way forward was "to establish a range of care management pilot schemes in order to test out and evaluate possible models for wider application"[38]. Staff were encouraged to put forward proposals for such pilots to the Care Management and Assessment Working Group.

However, the agreed pilot schemes were not fully established until April 1992, yet were expected to be evaluated by December 1992 in terms of the effectiveness of the assessment procedures used. This was so that recommendations could be made to the Social Services Committee on how best to implement assessment and care management within the Borough from April 1993[39]. Seven such schemes were introduced in April 1992, of which two were hospital based, two had a mental health focus, one focused on an adult services team and two related to specialist client groups.

One of the key tasks of the pilot schemes was to help develop the new assessment and eligibility criteria arrangements. Three stages of assessment were identified, namely initial screening, simple assessment and complex assessment[40]. From 1 April 1993, all new referrals would be 'screened' by access teams with support from specialist social work and occupational therapy teams to see whether the individual met the criteria for assessment. Such screening was intended to demonstrate where there was a requirement for a simple assessment for a one off or 'low intensity' service only. It would also identify the much smaller number of people who met the criteria for a complex needs assessment and would require a team of professionals across agencies to ensure a single multi-disciplinary assessment. A named social services worker from a relevant specialist team would be expected to coordinate such an assessment within a given timetable.

Crucial to the approach of the London Borough to assessment was the specification of eligibility for a complex assessment[41]. From the outset, these criteria were extensive but the clear emphasis was on clients in danger of entering expensive residential and nursing home care. The London Borough also placed a strong emphasis on levels of need, with the argument that those with high levels of need would have to be prioritised, given the limited resources made available to the local authority to implement the 'new' community care arrangements[42]. The assumption was also that the majority of those in high need would require a complex assessment.

In due course, both the different levels of the need and the eligibility criteria for a complex assessment were developed to relate specifically to older people[43]. With regard to levels of need, Figure 7.6 shows how severity of need was defined in terms of the tasks that the older person was unlikely to be able to complete. At the same time, eligibility for a complex assessment to consider admission to a nursing home was specified, as shown in Figure 7.7. The London Borough can be seen as having given considerable thought to care management and assessment, but the initial emphasis was very much about managing the costs of residential and nursing home entry.

It has been seen how County Council (B) placed a very high emphasis on its assessment arrangements as central to its commitment to provide user-centred community care. This was seen as requiring the complete

Figure 7.6: Defining levels of need (London Borough)[44]

High need	**Tasks unable to complete**
Assistance needed with personal care tasks every day, that is people who are unable to do two or more of the following:	• get in and out of bed; • eat and drink; • get to and use WC/commode; • get dressed; • wash hands and face; • may be incontinent.
Moderate need	**Tasks unable to complete**
Assistance needed several times a week, but less than every day, that is people who are unable to:	• bath/strip wash themselves; • do shopping; • cook meals; • do light household cleaning • are mildly confused.
Low need	
Potentially frail people who may need some preventative services.	

Figure 7.7: Eligibility criteria for admissions to nursing homes for older people (London Borough)[45]

- People who are ordinary residents of the Borough and are aged 75 and over.
- People whose physical abilities and understanding are such that they need constant care and supervision.
- People whose home circumstances are such that their independence cannot be maintained by relatives, carers, statutory or independent sector community services.
- People who need substantial assistance to manage basic daily living activities and personal care tasks, due to physical frailty.
- People whose needs require the attention of one or more carers, several times in any 24 hour period and nursing home care is considered the only option to alleviate stress for family or carers.
- People who need skilled nursing help because they have one or more chronic medical conditions (such as chronic obstructed airways disease, or cardio-vascular disease).
- People who need to live in a protected environment because otherwise they would be at serious risk, due to self-neglect, falling or fire hazard for example.
- People who are at risk of self-neglect, wandering or other harm as a result of dementia or confusion.
- People who have a long-standing mental disorder that cannot be appropriately managed in the home or community.

separation of purchaser and provider interests at the district office level so that care managers could focus solely upon the needs of the client (interview with Director of Social Services [B], 1990-93). As early as 1990, it had established a number of care management pilot schemes at the district level[46], and by April 1993 a common system of care management for both children and adults had been implemented across all the district offices of the social services department[47]. As with the London Borough, a clear system of eligibility was established with the authority being clear that care management is "how we will ration resources to ensure that care is provided to those in greatest need"[48]. The approach of County Council (B) also followed the London Borough in emphasising the need for different levels of assessment, with people initially being offered a simple assessment outside the care management system and only being "referred on ... for assessment if more serious problems emerge"[49].

The other crucial feature of the approach of this case study towards assessment and care management needs to be noted. A much greater level of financial devolution to care management teams existed in this authority compared to the London Borough (or the other two case studies). This was because care management was seen as the purchasing driver of the overall community care strategy. Care managers were expected to 'spot purchase' to meet the assessed needs of their clients, rather than to draw down from block contracts agreed at a much higher level in their authority. In this way it was hoped that services would develop in response to needs at the district level (interview with Director of Social Services [B], 1990-93).

More specifically, purchasing districts were allocated two types of budget:[50]

- budgets to cover direct costs (salaries, wages, establishment expenses, and so on) of the purchasing function;
- budgets to purchase services on behalf of clients (Service Purchasing Budgets) to be allocated by the client group.

The nominated officers responsible for these budgets were the purchaser district managers, although they could delegate further to individual care management teams subject to the joint accreditation and approval of the Director of Social Services and County Treasurer. Power to commit expenditure on any individual client was closely defined:

(i)   Care Team Managers up to £15,000 per annum;
(ii)   District Managers up to £30,000 per annum;
(iii) Assistant Directors up to £50,000 per annum[51].

This authority had a reputation for investment in information systems (Hoyes et al, 1992), but recognised that the logic of its radical approach would "require considerable investment" because "ultimately, the only solution is to have an integrated financial, contracting, purchasing and care management information system which will meet the County Council requirements"[52].

Senior managers in County Council (C) saw the community care reforms as offering an important opportunity to develop a more holistic rather than service driven approach to assessment:

> This notion of a holistic assessment that we have now, it wasn't there. So people somehow or other were referred, they were assessed by the home help organiser, or they were assessed by the meals on wheels organiser or they were referred to the district nurse for assessment or they were referred to a hospital. (interview with Principal Officer for the Elderly [C], 1989-93)

Yet at the same time, there was cynicism about the lack of resources available to implement such a holistic philosophy (interview with Director of Social Services [C], 1989-95), and this lack of resources ensured that "introducing the community care reforms ... meant introducing eligibility criteria" (interview with Director of Social Services [C], 1989-95).

What did this mean in practice? The previous section indicated how this authority was cautious about the advisability of adopting the kind of radical purchaser–provider split at the care management level of the kind adopted by County Council (B). However, it did define care management as covering "the tasks of assessment, care planning, implementation of plans, monitoring and review" and it did establish several care management pilot projects in 1991/92[53]. By March 1992, the social services department recognised that it still needed to complete work started in August 1991 on the establishment of "a standardised assessment across all client groups and agencies"[54]. It also realised that clarity on eligibility criteria would be crucial in the new system:

> The fundamental premise of all the community care developments is that the Social Services Department must assess what people need, not what services they could have. However, the committee will have to set out a policy framework for this needs level approach. This will have to cover the needs that will be assessed (the 'eligible needs'), the priority order of these eligible needs, and the criteria for gaining access to resources[55].

The amount of work required to establish the new purchasing/contracting approach and the practicalities of managing the transferred DSS monies meant that the work on eligibility was not expected to be concluded until just before the April 1993 deadline[56].

In many respects, the Metropolitan Authority adopted a similar approach to the London Borough and County Council (B) with regard to assessment and eligibility. First, it made a distinction between different levels of assessment:

a. *A simple assessment* for people with less complex needs. This would be undertaken using a standard format that could be used by staff from more than one agency. Services would be provided to those people meeting the criteria for eligibility for those services. All people would receive information about services available.
b. *A full assessment* would be provided for all people with complex needs, severe needs, or anyone requesting a full assessment. This would normally

be coordinated by a member of the Division, and would incorporate the participation of other agencies.

For either assessment, the individual person would be a full participant, and the outcome would be an agreed statement of need[57].

And then in terms of eligibility, it distinguished between high risk ("those at risk of serious harm and/or risk of admission to long-term care"[58]) and those at medium or low risk.

The view of this authority, as with the other three, was that public spending limits required very clear prioritisation based upon levels of need. More specifically, the following groups were deemed to be in the highest priority:

a. People who are alone and are unable through illness (physical or mental) or substantial disability (physical, sensory, mental or learning) to care for their own personal needs and who without support would be at substantial risk to life or serious injury.
b. People with the same illnesses, disabilities as above, but where their carer(s) are suffering serious stress and are at risk of illness/breakdown in their caring capacity.
c. People who, without statutory intervention, pose a serious threat to themselves or others.
d. People who are being or have been abused by others and are at serious threat of further abuse.
e. People who are occupying accommodation, such as a hospital bed or residential/nursing home place, but who could return home if specific services were provided, for example a stairlift[59].

The second level of priority were those in medium need who were seen as likely to fall into the highest need group if they did not receive at least some support services[60]. As part of this strategy, the Metropolitan Authority placed a high emphasis on information about services, including information for those individuals who fell outside the priority criteria for help from the local authority[61].

Conclusion

This chapter has profiled the efforts of the four case studies to begin the process of implementing the community care reforms in the early 1990s. It has confirmed the findings of earlier studies that local authorities found this to be an extremely complex and far-reaching task (Deakin, 1996;

Hoyes et al, 1994; Lewis and Glennerster, 1996; Wistow et al, 1994). Much of the initial energy may have been directed at how independent sector residential and nursing home places were to be purchased, but this chapter has also illustrated the far-reaching organisational changes being made within social services departments, in terms of care management, purchaser–provider splits and the growing emphasis on quality assurance.

It would seem that local authorities embraced quasi-markets as the way forward for community care for older people, despite initial reservations in some authorities. However, only five years later, a new Labour government would be complaining about the continued slowness of social services to use their lead agency role to deliver what older people really needed and wanted (see Chapter Two). The final chapter reflects on some of the reasons why this has happened. It also considers the key lessons and issues from the period 1971-93 which are most relevant to the challenge of providing health and welfare services for older people that are worthy of the 21st century.

Notes

[1] Social Services Committee (D), 16 March 1993 (Preparation for Implementation of Community Care).

[2] Social Services Committee (B), 23 June 1988 (The Griffiths Report: A Response).

[3] Social Services Committee (C), 10 September 1991 (Policy and Budget Plans, 1992-93 and 1993-94).

[4] Social Services Committee (A), 21 October 1992 (Community Care Implementation: Financial Implications).

[5] Social Services Committee (D), 15 October 1991 (Community Care Plan, 1992/93: Draft Plan).

[6] Social Services Committee (D), 16 March 1993 (Preparation for the Implementation of Community Care).

[7] Social Services Committee (D), 1 June 1992 (The Implementation of Community Care).

[8] Social Services Committee (A), 1 July 1991 (Proposed Re-organisation of the Social Services Department).

[9] Social Services Committee (A), 21 October 1992 (Establishing the Social Services Department's Commissioning Unit – Major Operational Issues).

[10] Social Services Committee (A), 19 January 1993 (Establishing the Quality Standards Section of the Quality Assurance and Planning Division).

[11] Social Services Committee (B), 21 November 1991 (Strategic Objectives: Establishing Care Management Teams in All District Offices).

[12] Ibid.

[13] *The Work of the Social Services Committee (B), April 1989 to March 1993: Report of Chairman*, 1 April 1993.

[14] Social Services Committee (B), 4 February 1993 (1990 NHS and Community Care Act/1989 Children Act: Committee/Management Strategy for 1993/94).

[15] Social Services Committee (B), 11 November 1992 (Quality Standards Directory).

[16] Social Services Committee (C), 15 December 1992 (Implementing Community Care: Review of Progress).

[17] Ibid.

[18] Social Services Committee (C), 22 September 1992 (1990 NHS and Community Care Act – Implementation Progress).

[19] Social Services Committee (D), 14 January 1991 (Preparation for Community Care).

[20] Ibid.

[21] Based on Appendix in Social Services Committee (D), 14 January 1991 (Preparation for Community Care).

[22] Social Services Committee (D), 28 May 1991 (Service Priorities, 1991-92).

[23] Social Services Committee (D), 1 June 1992 (Preparation for Implementation of Community Care).

[24] Social Services Committee (A), 21 October 1992 (Community Care Implementation).

[25] Ibid.

[26] Social Services Committee (A), 19 January 1993 (Commissioning Nursing/ Residential Home Placements).

[27] Ibid.

[28] Social Services Committee (B), 17 September 1992 (Quality Service Standards for Residential Care: Report on the Consultation).

[29] Ibid.

[30] Social Services Committee (C), 22 September 1992 (1990 NHS and Community Care Act – Implementation Progress).

[31] Ibid.

[32] Social Services Committee (C), 15 December 1992 (Implementing Community Care: Review of Progress).

[33] Social Services Committee (D), 16 March 1993 (Preparation for Implementation of Community Care).

[34] Ibid.

[35] Social Services Committee (D), 2 June 1993 (The Implementation of Community Care).

[36] Ibid.

[37] Social Services Committee (A), 8 April 1991 (Review of the Key Strategic Issues for Social Services, 1990/91 and Proposed Service Plans for 1991/92).

[38] Social Services Committee (A), 1 July 1991 (Community Care: Progress to Date).

[39] Social Services Committee (A), 21 January 1992 (Community Care – Care Management Pilot Projects).

[40] Social Services Committee (A), 21 October 1992 (Community Care Implementation: Care Management and Assessment).

[41] Ibid.

[42] Ibid.

[43] Social Services Committee (A), 19 January 1993 (Criteria for Eligibility for Services (Adults) Policy).

[44] Ibid.

[45] Social Services Committee (A), 21 October 1992 (Community Care Implementation – Criteria for Nursing Homes and the Development and Eligibility Criteria for Services).

[46] Social Services Committee (B), 17 September 1990 ('Caring for People': The 1990 NHS and Community Care Act).

[47] Social Services Committee (B), 17 September 1992 (NHS and Community Care Act: Progress Report).

---

[48] Social Services Committee (B), 11 November 1992 (Quality Standards Directory).

[49] Ibid.

[50] Social Services Committee (B), 4 February 1993 (Care Management Teams: Budget Management Rules).

[51] Ibid.

[52] Social Services Committee (B), 17 September 1992 (NHS and Community Care Act: Progress Report).

[53] Social Services Committee (C), 3 March 1992 (Implementing the Community Care Act).

[54] Ibid.

[55] Ibid.

[56] Social Services Committee (C), 15 December 1992 (Implementing Community Care, Review of Progress).

[57] Social Services Committee (D), 14 January 1991 (Preparation for Community Care).

[58] Ibid.

[59] Social Services Committee (D), 19 January 1993 (Community Care Implementation).

[60] Ibid.

[61] Social Services Committee (D), 1 June 1992 (Preparation for Implementation of Community Care).

EIGHT

Developing community care for the future: lessons and issues from the past

Introduction

Chapter Two set out the modernisation agenda of the 1997-2001 Labour government and its implications for community care. A Labour government was re-elected in 2001 with a clear mandate to continue its modernisation agenda for public services. This last chapter therefore reflects on lessons and issues from this study in terms of the challenge to develop further community care in the new millennium.

A lack of policy direction? A lack of priority?

The period, 1971 to the mid-1980s, was characterised by a lack of priority and policy direction with regard to health and welfare services for older people. It could be argued that this situation was changed by the quasi-market reforms in community care of the early 1990s and was further influenced by the modernisation policies of recent Labour governments. More specifically, many would feel that this situation has been transformed through the establishment of a National Service Framework for Older People (DoH, 2001b), which sets out eight standards relating to age discrimination, person-centred care, intermediate care, general hospital care, stroke, falls, mental health in old age and health promotion (see Figure 8.1). It is hard to argue that we lack a comprehensive policy direction.

This is true, but only to a limited extent for three reasons. First, there is still no consolidated legal framework relating to services for older people equivalent to the 1989 Children Act. Instead, discussions about the health and social care divide and the so called 'Berlin Wall' still have to refer back to the 1948 National Assistance Act and the introduction of the concept of being 'in need of care and attention'. Equally, the provision of

Figure 8.1: The eight standards of the national service framework

Standard 1: Rooting out age discrimination
NHS services will be provided, regardless of age, on the basis of clinical need alone. Social care services will not use age in their eligibility criteria or policies, to restrict access to available services.

Standard 2: Person-centred care
NHS and social care services will treat older people as individuals and enable them to make choices about their own care. This will be achieved through the single assessment process, integrated commissioning arrangements and integrated provision of services, including community equipment and continence services.

Standard 3: Intermediate care
Older people will have access to a new range of intermediate care services at home, or in designated care settings, to promote their independence by providing enhanced services from the NHS and councils to prevent ·
unnecessary hospital admission and effective rehabilitation services to enable early discharge from hospital and to prevent premature or unnecessary admission to long-term residential care.

Standard 4: General hospital care
Older people's care in hospital will be delivered through appropriate specialist care and by hospital staff who have the right set of skills to meet their needs.

Standard 5: Stroke
The NHS will take action to prevent strokes, working in partnership with other agencies where appropriate. People who are thought to have had a stroke will have access to diagnostic services, be treated appropriately by a specialist stroke service, and subsequently, with their carers, participate in a multidisciplinary programme of secondary prevention and rehabilitation.

Standard 6: Falls
The NHS working in partnership with councils, will take action to prevent falls and reduce resultant fractures or other injuries in their populations of older people. Older people who have fallen will receive effective treatment and rehabilitation and, with their carers, receive advice on prevention, through a specialised falls service.

Standard 7: Mental health in older people
Older people who have mental health problems will have access to integrated mental health services, provided by the NHS and councils to ensure effective diagnosis, treatment and support, for them and for their carers.

Standard 8: The promotion of health and active life in older age
The health and well being of older people will be promoted through a coordinated programme of action led by the NHS with support from councils.

Source: DoH (2001b, pp 12-14)

social care services in the community relates to a variety of different Acts dating back to the late 1960s and early 1970s.

The second point is that the government rejected the main proposal of the *Royal Commission on Long-Term Care* (Sutherland Report, 1999) that all personal care should be free. Although this has been justified in terms of the need to invest in new services rather than subsidise old ones, not all commentators are convinced (see Chapter Two). It is true that substantial additional money is being invested in intermediate care, but it is doubtful if all the eight standards of the national framework can possibly be met within allocated resources. As such, another continuity with the past can be identified, namely the tendency of central government to set unrealistic objectives for community care services for older people, which was one of the main complaints of the Griffiths Report (1988).

The final point is that even if one argues that the financial investment in intermediate care is impressive, it would still seem that the central motivation and dominant political concern is not the quality of life of older people but rather bed blockage. The NHS Plan makes the bold assertion that "by 2004 we will end widespread bed blocking" (Secretary of State for Health, 2000a, p 102). It is hard to avoid the conclusion that what is being demanded is the speedy removal of older people from hospital. One hopes this will occur through a greater investment in genuine rehabilitation services, rather than just under the guise of rehabilitation. It would be too easy for much private residential and nursing home accommodation to be redefined as short-term rehabilitation beds, even though they might often lead on only to long-term care in the same institution. This might prove very tempting given the complexities of developing more imaginative approaches, such as multi-agency community-based rehabilitation schemes (Thomas and Means, 2000).

In the past we have explored the reasons for the traditional neglect of services for older people and considered such factors as political economy (older people have neither a productive nor reproductive role in a capitalist society), the desire of the state to maximise the input of informal carers and stereotypes about ageing, illness and death (Means and Smith, 1998b). This book has provided numerous examples of such neglect in the 1971-93 period. A positive reading of government plans and proposals would suggest a final break with the 'Cinderella Services' tag initially labelled in the 1950s (Means and Smith, 1998a). However, this would be a very generous reading of likely outcomes and it is far from clear that this will turn out to be the case in practice.

Paying for long-term care? The role of long-term care?

One of the elements of neglect considered in Means and Smith (1998b) is the role of institutions as a warning to others. This was certainly true at the time of the Poor Law:

> The workhouse represented the ultimate sanction. The fact that comparatively few people came to be admitted did not detract from the power of its negative image, an image that was sustained by the accounts that circulated about the harsh treatment and separation of families that admission entailed. The success of 'less eligibility' in deterring the able-bodied and others from seeking relief relied heavily on the currency of such images. (Parker, 1988, p 9)

However, it has been argued by Townsend that this role was subsequently taken up by the local authority residential home:

> Residential homes for the elderly serve functions for the wider society and not only for their inmates. While accommodating only a tiny percentage of the elderly population, they symbolise the dependence of the elderly and legitimate their lack of access to equality of status. (Townsend, 1986, p 32)

Could our four case study authorities be accused of colluding with this type of situation?

This would seem an unreasonable accusation and hard to sustain from the evidence presented in this book. However, Chapter Four showed how local authorities were extremely slow to begin to focus on the quality of life of older residents and it was only the publication of *Home life* (Avebury, 1984), and the subsequent emphasis by central government on its relevance to local authority homes, which seemed to stimulate social services authorities to address such issues. It is also true that the level of investment in homes was never adequate enough to deliver on the original aspirations of those who drafted the 1948 National Assistance Act. Instead of residential hotels, the legacy of Poor Law institutions and Poor Law staff drifted on, and was never fully overcome. Chapter Four demonstrated how far into our study period outdated and inadequate buildings were still commonplace and justified on the grounds that they were for older people who had never been used to anything better. More subtle than this was the failure, because of public expenditure pressures, to reinvest in residential homes built in the late 1960s and early 1970s. It was *Home life* that once again exposed the inadequacy of much of what was available as direct provision by local authorities.

Nevertheless, 'the EPH wars' (interview with Director of Social Services [C], 1988-95) profiled in Chapter Four, suggested that older people as well as opposition councillors and trades unionists, often objected not only to home closure but also to the transfer of homes into the independent sector. This suggests that most local authority homes were 'homes' to their residents and not just institutions.

A key continuity with the past is certainly the capacity of long-term care to dominate debates about community care at both the local and national level. In the early 1970s, the focus was on building local authority homes. From the late 1980s the emphasis became the need to update, close or transfer these homes. It was also about the need to 'cap' the mushrooming cost of social security payments for those in independent sector residential and nursing care. The broad vision of both *Making a reality of community care* (Audit Commission, 1986) and the Griffiths Report (1988) was translated by government into a concern to cash-limit public expenditure on independent homes through a transfer of responsibilities to local authorities.

This last point suggests that it is the cost of institutional care rather than its symbolic importance that is the dominant concern of governments. One reason for the shifting boundary between health and social care, outlined in Chapters Four and Five, was that NHS care is free while social care can be means tested and charged for. This is also the most likely explanation for the rejection by the present government of the proposal for free personal care from the Royal Commission (Sutherland Report, 1999), despite the desire to break down the 'Berlin Wall' between health and social care through the establishment of care trusts (see below).

What is the boundary between health and social care? What is the future of social services?

It has just been argued that a central explanation for the shifting boundary between health and social care is the fact that health care is free and social care can be charged for. Chapter Five profiled in detail some of the tensions that were created from the resultant decline in continuing care beds in the NHS and the increased level of dependency in local authority residential homes. The trend of declining continuing care beds was, of course, massively speeded up by the growth of independent sector nursing homes. Equally important for social services was the earlier discharge of older people from hospital with the resultant increased pressures upon community services. Joint finance and joint planning may have enabled the development of some innovative services, but Chapter Five demonstrated how they often served only to increase tensions between health and social care.

The Griffiths Report (1988) and the subsequent White Paper (DoH, 1989a) led, of course, to a further boundary redefinition through social services departments taking over many of the assessment and funding responsibilities for those in independent nursing home care. The logic of this has been challenged:

> Despite the claim that the responsibilities of the NHS are unchanged, nursing home care is apparently now viewed as social care, not health. Is this contradictory, or are we to accept that there is a real distinction between those needing nursing home care for reasons of ill health and those needing it for other reasons? Surely this is playing *Alice in Wonderland* games with words and semantics. (Henwood, 1992, p 28)

However, at another level the logic was only too clear. The boundary had been redefined, yet again, in the direction of social care embracing ever more dependent people in order to control the public expenditure costs of older people with health and social care problems.

Another important continuity with the present is how the period 1971–93 saw social services taking on ever greater responsibilities but without an equivalent transfer of resources from the National Health Service. Chapter Five showed how even joint finance required social services to 'pick up' the tab after the initial grant period. Resultant arguments and tensions between health and social services agencies were only to be expected, and, in historical perspective, it could be argued that actual relationships were often much better than could reasonably have been expected.

From this perspective it is probably unfair to talk of a 'Berlin Wall'. However, in so far as one has developed, this book illustrates how its construction goes back a long way and the reasons for its development can be easily explained. Recent Labour governments have expressed a determination to destroy once and for all this supposed wall and to insist on 'joined up solutions' from health and social care to meet the needs of older people. Chapter Two explained how a duty of partnership was created through the 1999 Health Act and how joint working is to be further fostered through care trusts. Care trusts make most sense if one accepts that there is no clear distinction to be made between the health and social care components of personal care as proposed by the Royal Commission (Sutherland Report, 1999). However, the government has of course responded to the majority view of the Commission by stressing that such a distinction does exist. As a result, the new care trusts will have to explain to their clients why some elements of their personal care are free (that is, community nursing) but others are not (that is, home care).

It is open to doubt whether the government can sustain this position.

Already, the Scottish Parliament has made a commitment to introduce free personal care and this was supported for the rest of the United Kingdom by the Liberal Democrats (Liberal Democrats, 2001) in their 2001 General Election manifesto. It is, of course, quite possible that the next decade will see pressure mount in the direction of means testing and charging for both health and social care community services, although this is an approach that would receive virtually no public support at the moment. However, it could be argued that the Labour government elected in 2001 may be very willing to push health and social care services in this direction (see below).

As explained in Chapter Two, many social workers now see no future for traditional social services departments (Downey, 2001). However, government guidance on care trusts stress that they are not about to take over social services departments (DoH, 2001a). It would appear that they will essentially be NHS bodies in which accountability back to democratically elected councillors will be extremely limited. The community care landscape for older people is about to be changed dramatically and it is hard to avoid the conclusion that the lead agency role for social services as argued for by the Griffiths Report (1988) is in the process of being terminated.

This is a high risk strategy for at least two reasons. First, the history of community care services warns us of the deleterious impact of reorganisations on service delivery because of what is often called implementation deficit (Pressman and Wildavsky, 1973). This book covers the early period of disruption associated with the establishment of unified social services departments in April 1971 and concludes with the extensive community care changes (see Chapter Seven) demanded by the 1990 NHS and Community Care Act. In between, there have been numerous major reorganisations of the National Health Service and significant changes to local authority boundaries and levels of responsibility. It is hard to avoid the conclusion that the one consequence of this is that the focus often becomes structures rather than the quality of services on the ground. In fairness to the Griffiths Report (1988), it argued for radical reform but in a way designed to minimise formal organisational change of the National Health Service and social services departments. The government has clearly decided that the Griffiths approach has failed to break down the 'Berlin Wall' and that more fundamental change is required. Is this negative view justified? And will possible future gains justify the short to medium term problems of implementation deficit?

Linked to this, the second reason why care trusts are a high risk strategy is that social services departments have made a reasonable success of their lead agency role in community care when judged by the criteria of the quality of services delivered on the ground, despite the resource limitations. *Modernising social services* (see Chapter Two) claimed that "social services are often failing to provide the support that people should expect" (DoH, 1998a, p 5) and yet this is not fully backed up by the research evidence. Indeed, the contribution from the Department of Health by Warburton and McCracken (1999) to the *Royal Commission on Long-Term care* (Sutherland Report, 1999) acknowledged this. The authors reviewed research commissioned by the Department of Health against the question of whether older people were getting a better service compared to 6 to 10 years previously. They concluded that the answer was clear-cut, since in 1998 compared to the early 1990s:

- the number of people aged 65 and over in residential care has stabilised;
- spending on residential care and nursing homes has been brought under control;
- many older people are being assessed in order to determine the type of long-term care they should receive;
- there is evidence that care packages for older people living at home are more efficiently meeting needs, and that services are benefiting a wider range of people;
- there is a more planned approach to the social care of older people, facilitated by the widespread development of care management procedures;
- area-based qualified social workers, working as care managers, are now more closely involved in the assessments and care plans of older people;
- the views, circumstances and needs of carers are more recognised and taken into account (Warburton and McCracken, 1999, pp 25-6).

Such a perspective has also been backed up by Bauld et al (2000) in their review of the findings of the Evaluating Community Care for Elderly People research project of the University of Kent's Personal Social Services Research Unit. They concluded that "the greater emphasis on care management and planning has resulted in scarce resources being targeted more effectively than hitherto towards those older people with the greatest needs, and there is clear evidence that this resulted in tangible benefits for users" (p 388). Chapter Three argued that the 1980s and early 1990s demonstrated much more talk about targeting and prioritisation than real change. Bauld et al (2000) demonstrate how dramatically this had changed by the end of the millennium.

From this perspective, tensions with health and failures to invest in prevention and rehabilitation can be seen as the by-product of "a system where resources in relation to needs have been tightly constrained for many years" (Bauld et al, 2000, p 388), rather than the inability of social services to manage change. The main argument for the establishment of care trusts might be simply that this is the only way to generate more resources for community care for older people since this makes them part of the National Health Service rather than the responsibility of local authorities (Means et al, 2000). Yet it seems more likely that it is the temptation of the organisational fix that is the main government driver and this is a very high risk strategy indeed. The integration of "health and social services into one organisation" may be "a logical progression" (Gillam, 2001, pp 21-2), but it is one where primary care itself is close to reorganisation chaos.

Planning versus markets? Mixed economy or privatisation?

In his recent review of government policy initiatives in social care, Hudson (2000) has argued:

> ... the real change is not so much in what is done, so much as the way in which it is done ... social services will in future be subject to an unprecedented degree of central command and surveillance with far reaching consequences for their future existence, let alone direction. (p 237)

Chapters Three and Four illustrated how both Conservative and Labour governments attempted central command during the 1970s through establishing "priorities for health and personal social services" (DHSS, 1976b), while Chapters Six and Seven looked at the Thatcherite plan to put more emphasis on markets and competition.

It would be an error to interpret Labour government policy as being anti markets and competition, since competition is a core principle of Best Value (see Chapter Two). However, this is a government with a clear view about the need to enforce major changes in health and welfare provision, and it believes in doing this through establishing targets, and then often paying (or punishing) through results. Strong performance can lead to additional resources – poor performance can lead to the removal of the authority to run or be responsible for future service development.

This stress on targets can be well illustrated by the *National service*

Figure 8.2: Intermediate care implementation plans

The NHS and councils should, in line with the national guidance:

• agree a three year implementation plan for intermediate care, as part of the
  Local Action Plan and Joint Investment Plan, with arrangements for
  systematic monitoring and review focusing on:

  - responding to or averting a crisis – including, for every PCG/T area, a
    clear strategy for preventing avoidable acute hospital admissions;

  - rehabilitation and recovery – to include discharge/rehabilitation planning
    at the earliest possible opportunity during an acute hospital admission.
    Every PCG/T area to develop an appropriate range of services to meet
    local needs;

  - preventing unnecessary or premature admission to residential care –
    ensuring that early investment is targeted at service users at highest risk
    and that care plans clearly identify any potential for rehabilitation;

• ensure that the plan addresses the service, organisational and personal
  development needs of the new intermediate care teams.

Source: DoH (2001b, p 49)

framework for older people (DoH, 2001b). In terms of intermediate care
(only one of eight standards in the framework), the NHS and local
authorities have to establish implementation plans at the local level (see
Figure 8.2) in order to achieve ambitious milestones at the national level
(see Figure 8.3). The 1990 Act reforms were based on a critique of local
authority performance in community care. As Hudson (2000) indicates,
Labour governments have taken new surveillance powers way beyond
the 1990 Act in the hope of improving the performance of local authorities
and especially the quality of their working with the health service (see
Chapter Five). However, one consequence of this is that central
government might come to be held much more accountable than in the
past by the general public for the quality of both welfare as well as health
services for older people. What happens if these ambitious targets are not
met, partly as a result of implementation deficits caused through the
establishment of care trusts? In many parts of the country, it will no
longer be relevant to blame social services departments and local
government.

In the 'mainstream' health service, the government has shown an
increased tendency to turn to the private sector and private sector finance
as a crucial mechanism for speeding up modernisation change, as stressed
in its General Election manifesto:

> ... specially built surgical units – managed by the NHS or the private
> sector – will guarantee shorter waiting times – we will use the spare
> capacity in private sector hospitals, treating NHS patients free of charge,

where high standards and value for money are guaranteed. (Labour
Party, 2001, p 22)

It is, therefore, certain that the Labour government re-elected in 2001
will remain committed to a mixed economy of social care with a strong
emphasis on the service delivery role of both the voluntary and private
sectors. The deep roots of this mixed economy were traced in Chapter
Six, including the growing emphasis on service agreements linked to
social services departments. The period since 1993 has seen a sustained
expansion of social care markets for older people across both long-term
care and domiciliary services (Knapp et al, 2001). As Player and Pollock
(2001) put it with regard to long-term care, "government policies show
no enthusiasm for returning to public provision or accountability, or to
the principle of collective risk pooling through social insurance" (p 252).

But how far might privatisation in community care be pushed?
Certainly, the Labour government believes in means testing for personal
care, as already discussed, although it needs to be remembered that the

Figure 8.3: Intermediate care milestones

July 2001	Local health and social care systems to have designated a jointly appointed intermediate care coordinator in at least each health authority area; to have agreed the framework for patient/user and carer involvement; and to have completed the baseline mapping exercise.
January 2002	Local health and social care systems to have agreed the joint investment plan for 2002/03.
March 2002	At least 1,500 additional intermediate care beds compared with the 1999/2000 baseline.
	At least 40,000 additional people receiving intermediate care services that promote rehabilitation and supported discharge compared with the 1999/2000 baseline.
	At least 20,000 additional people receiving intermediate care that prevents unnecessary hospital admission compared with the 1999/2000 baseline.
March 2004	At least 5,000 additional intermediate care beds and 1,700 non-residential intermediate care places compared with the 1999/2000 baseline.
	At least 150,000 additional people receiving intermediate care services that promote rehabilitation and supported discharge compared with the 1999/2000 baseline.
	At least 70,000 additional people receiving intermediate care that prevents unnecessary hospital admission compared with the 1999/2000 baseline.

Source: DoH (2001b, pp 49-50)

principle of charging for domiciliary services can be traced back to the 1940s (see Chapter Three). Equally, those older people with resources who are deemed to be a low priority for help from social services are now increasingly in a position to buy personal care from the private market, not only through long-term care, but also through agencies providing 'support at home' services.

However, it would seem unfair to claim that the Labour government has any intention to remove or dramatically reduce extensive public expenditure on community care for older people, even if the better off will be encouraged to self-provide and even if there is an ever greater reliance on the private sector both in terms of the delivery of services and through public-private financial partnerships. As such, it is perhaps best to see the system as continuing to be a quasi-market (see Chapter Seven), but one that the government has decided to manipulate through the Health Service rather than through local authorities.

Economic imperatives

The modernisation agenda is being funded as a result of a period of economic prosperity and low inflation. Not only are public expenditure commitments likely to be reduced should this situation change, but the impact of this is especially likely to be felt by older people as very high consumers of public welfare. The political economy perspective (Phillipson, 1982, 1998; Walker, 1981) has always recognised the marginal nature of older people in market economies, a group most of whom are no longer in the labour market, nor involved in the day-to-day upbringing of children.

The early 1970s saw the speed at which a commitment to rapid public expenditure growth could be translated into major cutbacks. The sterling and oil crises were very much the start of a recognition of the global nature of the world economy and how globalisation had the power to restrict and shape developments in individual nation states. The trend seems certain to continue and should warn the reader to look for the economic imperatives behind 'modernisation' in the same way that could be found behind 'Thatcherism'.

One implication for older people is that the emphasis by government on the need to maximise informal or family care is likely to continue, despite the changing nature of family relationships in present day Britain (Phillipson et al, 2001), and the challenge offered by an older population soon to expand rapidly (Evandrou, 1997). The national service framework may offer a new vision, but it is a vision rooted in many of the same assumptions that can be traced back at least to the reconstruction debates at the end of the Second World War (Means and Smith, 1998a).

Nothing changes? Everything changes?

In our earlier study (Means and Smith, 1998a), we quoted the historian Anne Digby for her crucial insight into the value of an historical perspective on present policy debates:

> The lesson of history is that it does not repeat itself precisely, yet, on a broader front, certain policy issues, dilemmas, problems and choices do recur in social welfare. To forget the past record of these events is to force each generation to relearn what should already be known, and thus make future developments less satisfactory than they might be. Equally undesirable, however, has been the tendency in some quarters to manufacture mythical virtues which present policy can seek to emulate. Through each of these historical tendencies, current debate on social welfare is made less informed and cogent. (Digby, 1989, p 1)

In other words, it would be completely wrong to interpret this book, and especially this chapter, as saying 'nothing changes'. Rather, it is seeking to show how right Digby was to stress the recurrence of certain policy issues, dilemmas, problems and choices, irrespective of the locality under study or the political hue of the central government. If nothing else, we hope that this book has demonstrated that the golden age of community care in the 1970s was a myth, and yet equally it was never the disaster claimed by so many on the Right.

The years 1971-93 covered a period that saw significant changes as well as continuities. One of these relates to language and terminology. EMI (Elderly Mentally Infirm) homes have become homes for Elderly People with Dementia. Grants have become service agreements. And so on. It would be nice to be able to argue that 'the elderly' had become 'individual older people' during the study period. Chapter Four suggested some progress in this area with the growth of consumer rights in residential care, but it would be wrong to over emphasise progress in this direction.

It is also possible to identify the emergence of new discourses. Race and ethnicity were completely missing from the discourse of the 1939-71 period (Means and Smith, 1998a), but are more clearly present in the second half of the 1971-93 timeframe. In this book, this development has been mainly addressed in terms of the voluntary sector in the London Borough (see Chapter Six), but similar debates were also found in the

Metropolitan Authority and in at least one of the two County Councils. Whether the level of debate was adequate and whether it led to improved service provision for black and minority ethnic older people is a complex issue to address.

Another important change has been the emergence of the private sector as the dominant provider in long-term care and a key provider of home-based personal care (Laing and Saper, 1999). It needs to be remembered how the nature of that private sector has changed from that of the classic cottage industry of family run single homes (Phillips et al, 1988) to one "increasingly dominated by generic, often publicly-quoted multi-national corporations" (Player and Pollock, 2001, p 231). The growth of this sector has been supported not only by the availability of public subsidy, but also by the massive expansion of housing wealth amongst older people. In the early 1970s, it was still far more common for older people to rent rather than to own their properties but owner occupation is now by far the most common tenure in later life (Heywood et al, 2001). The resources and aspirations of older people in 2001 are very different from those of older people in 1971.

The availability of social networks and social support for older people has also changed quite dramatically, as demonstrated in the research by Phillipson et al (2001). This stressed the continued importance of kinship but in a context where relationships are now much more dispersed and fragmented, and where the family life of older people is more varied as a result of "reflecting distinct types of urban change, migration histories, social class and age relations" (p 254). However, despite these changes, a key continuity between this study and the previous one (Means and Smith, 1998a) is the emphasis by government on the need to encourage the maximum input from informal carers as a way of controlling the public expenditure costs of personal care for older people. In the 1950s, the fear was that the availability of home care from the state would discourage family care. By the early 1990s, the emphasis was on targeted support for carers, increasingly seen as the spouse rather than the next generation. Perhaps, the next stage will be a renewed emphasis on friends and neighbours as part of community regeneration.

The final change relates to the importance of the technological revolution. As we have argued elsewhere, care management and the management of the mixed economy depend on the creative use of computer-based information systems (Means and Smith, 1998b). This will be equally true of the common assessment approach for older people across health and social services agencies proposed by the national service framework (DoH, 2001b). And yet research evidence is that social services have often made only limited investment in such resources (Hoyes and Means, 1994) and that existing information systems are often poorly coordinated (Qureshi, 1999). Social services are left trying to deliver community care for the 21st century with an infrastructure that is too often little changed from the 1980s. This is perhaps another factor that will push the Labour government to a care trust 'solution' for community care for older people, since it might prove the easiest way to move towards integrated information systems across health and social services agencies.

With regard to information technology, Hoggett stressed over a decade ago that:

> ... whilst contemporary processes of modernisation may be technologically driven, they are not technologically determined. A variety of social choices are possible within the frame provided by a given techno-managerial paradigm. (1990, p 15)

At this point, it becomes crucial to guard against one's own capacity to construct past 'golden ages'. One of us as a local authority social worker in the mid-1970s remembers the energy and enthusiasm of the period. This was also supported by one of the Directors of Social Services interviewed who claimed "the contrast between the enthusiasm, commitment and optimism of the early 1970s and the situation today is quite marked" (interview with Director of Social Services [A], 1971-80). However, this is a dangerous train of thought to follow because it begins to deny the possibilities of influence outlined by Hoggett. We need to believe that existing and future cohorts of health and welfare professionals will wish to work with older people on building a positive vision of community care (Means and Smith, 1998b). There are real dangers in the modernisation agenda, such as excessive surveillance, an over reliance on the private sector and an ill thought out radical restructuring of the health and social care boundary. But there are also real possibilities in terms of the reinvestment in services.

In the early 1970s, new investment was often 'wasted' on very traditional residential services. Let us make sure that the same mistake is not made in the early years of the 21st century.

References

Audit Commission (1985) *Managing social services for the elderly more effectively*, London: HMSO.

Audit Commission (1986) *Making a reality of community care*, London: HMSO.

Avebury, K. (1984) *Home life: A code of practice for residential care*, London: Centre for Policy on Ageing.

Baldwin, S. and Lunt, N. (1996) *Charging ahead: The development of local authority charging policies for community care*, Bristol/York: The Policy Press/Joseph Rowntree Foundation.

Baldwin, S. and Parker, G. (1989) 'The Griffiths Report on community care', in M. Brenton and C. Ungerson (eds) *Social Policy Review, 1988-89*, London: Longman, pp 143-65.

Bartlett, W., Propper, C., Wilson, D. and Le Grand, J. (eds) (1994) *Quasi-markets in the welfare state*, Bristol: SAUS Publications.

Bauld, L., Chesterman, J., Davies, B., Judge, K. and Mangalore, R. (2000) *Caring for older people: An assessment of community care in the 1990s*, Aldershot: Ashgate.

Beveridge, W. (1948) *Voluntary action*, London: Allen and Unwin.

Biggs, S. (1990/91) 'Consumers, care management and inspection: obscuring social deprivation and need', *Critical Social Policy*, Issue 30, pp 23-8.

Bosanquet, N. (1978) *A future for old age*, London: Temple Smith.

Boucher Report (1957) *Survey of services available to the chronic sick and elderly, 1954-55*, London: HMSO.

Brooke, E. (1950) 'The aged in hospital and at home', in *Welfare Problems of Old People*, Fifth National Conference of NOPWC, London: NCSS.

Brown, R.G.S. (1979) *Reorganising the National Health Service*, Oxford: Basil Blackwell and Martin Robertson.

Burns, A., Howard, R. and Pettit, W. (1997) *Alzheimer's disease: A medical companion*, Oxford: Blackwell Press.

Chetwynd, M., Ritchie, J., Reith, M. and Howard, M. (1996) *The cost of care: The impact of charging policy on the lives of disabled people*, Bristol/York: The Policy Press/Joseph Rowntree Foundation.

Davies, B. (1981) 'Strategic goals and piecemeal innovation: adjusting to the new balance of needs and resources', in E. Goldberg and S. Hatch (eds) *A new look at the personal social services*, London: Policy Studies Institute, pp 46-67.

Deakin, N. (1996) 'The devils in the detail: some reflections on contracting for social care for voluntary organisations', *Social Policy and Administration*, vol 30, no 1, pp 20-38.

Deputy Prime Minister (1998) *Modern local government: In touch with the people*, Cm 4014, London: The Stationery Office.

DETR (Department of the Environment, Transport and the Regions) (1998) *Modernising local government: Improving local services through Best Value*, London: DETR.

DETR (1999) *Implementing Best Value: A consultative paper on draft guidance*, London: DETR.

DHSS (Department of Health and Social Security) (1971) *Help in the home: Section 13 of the Health Services and Public Health Act*, LAC Circular (71) 53, London: DHSS.

DHSS (1972) *Local authority social services ten year development plans 1973-1983*, Circular 35/72, London: DHSS.

DHSS (1975) *Local authority expenditure in 1976/77 – forward planning*, LAC Circular (75) 10, London: DHSS.

DHSS (1976a) *Prevention and health: Everybody's business*, London: HMSO.

DHSS (1976b) *Priorities for health and personal social services in England: A consultative document*, London: HMSO.

DHSS (1976c) *The elderly and the personal social services*, London: DHSS.

DHSS (1976d) *A lifestyle for the elderly*, London: DHSS.

DHSS (1977) *Priorities in the health and social services: The way forward*, London: HMSO.

DHSS (1978a) *A happier old age: A discussion document on elderly people in our society*, London: HMSO.

DHSS (1978b) *Collaboration in community care: A discussion document*, London: HMSO.

DHSS (1981a) *Care in action: A handbook of policies and priorities for the health and personal social services in England*, London: HMSO.

DHSS (1981b) *Care in the community: A consultative document on moving resources for care in England*, London: DHSS.

DHSS (1981c) *Growing older*, Cm 8173, London: HMSO.

DHSS (1981d) *The respective roles of the general acute and geriatric sectors in the care of the elderly hospital patient*, London: DHSS.

DHSS (1981e) *The report of a study on the acute hospital sector*, London: HMSO.

DHSS (1983) *Health service development: Care in the community and joint finance*, Health Circular (83)6 and Local Authority Circular (83)5, London: DHSS.

DHSS (1985) *Progress in partnership: Report of a working group on joint planning*, London: DHSS.

DHSS (1986a) *Neighbourhood nursing: A focus for care*, Cumberlege Report, London: HMSO.

DHSS (1986b) *Primary health care: An agenda for discussion*, London: HMSO.

DHSS (1987) *Promoting better health: The government's programme for improving primary health care*, Cm 249, London: HMSO.

DHSS and the Welsh Office (1979) *Patients first: Consultative paper on the structure and management of the National Health Service in England and Wales*, London: HMSO.

Digby, A. (1989) *British welfare policy: Workhouse to workfare*, London: Faber and Faber.

Dobson, F. (1997) Paper presented at the annual conference of the NHS Confederation, Brighton, 25 June.

DoH (Department of Health) (1989a) *Caring for people: Community care in the next decade and beyond*, Cm 849, London: HMSO.

DoH (1989b) *Working for patients*, Cm 555, London: HMSO.

DoH (1990) *Community care in the next decade and beyond: Policy guidance*, London: HMSO.

DoH (1991) *Purchase of service: Practice guidance and practice materials*, London: HMSO.

DoH (1992) *Memorandum on the financing of community care arrangements after April 1993*, London: DoH, 2 October.

DoH (1997) *The new NHS: Modern, dependable*, Cm 3807, London: The Stationery Office.

DoH (1998a) *Modernising social services – promoting independence, improving protection, raising standards*, Cm 4169, London: The Stationery Office.

DoH (1998b) *Our healthier nation: A contract for health*, Cm 3852, London: The Stationery Office.

DoH (1999) *Saving lives: Our healthier nation*, Cm 3486, London: The Stationery Office.

DoH (2001a) *Care trusts: Emerging framework*, London: DoH, March.

DoH (2001b) *National Service Framework for older people*, London: DoH, March.

DoH/DETR (Department of the Environment, Transport and the Regions) (1999) *Health Act 1999 – modern partnerships for the people*, letter to health and social care agencies, 8 September.

DoH/Social Services Inspectorate (1991a) *Care management and assessment: Managers guide*, London: HMSO.

DoH/Social Services Inspectorate (1991b) *Care management and assessment: Practitioners guide*, London: HMSO.

Dominelli, L. and Hoogvelt, A. (1996) 'Globalisation and the technocratisation of social work', *Critical Social Policy*, vol 16, no 2, pp 45-62.

Downey, R. (2001) 'In poll position', *Community Care*, 31 May-6 June, pp 20-2.

Driver, S. and Martell, L. (2000) 'Left, Right and the third way', *Policy & Politics*, vol 28, no 2, pp 147-62.

DSS (Department of Social Security) (1998) *A new contract for welfare: Principles into practice*, Cm 4101, London: The Stationery Office.

Enthoven, A. (1985) *Reflections on the management of the National Health Service*, London: Nuffield Provincial Hospitals Trust.

Evandrou, M. (ed) (1997) *Baby boomers: What future when we retire?*, London: Age Concern.

Firth Report (1987) *Public support for residential care*, Joint Central and Local Government Working Party, London: DHSS.

Flynn, N. (1989) 'The New Right and social policy', *Policy & Politics*, vol 17, no 2, pp 97-110.

Geddes, M. and Martin, S. (2000) 'The policy and politics of Best Value: Comments, crosscurrents and undercurrents in the new regime', *Policy & Politics*, vol 28, no 3, pp 379-95.

Gillam, S. (2001) 'Perpetual revolution: a stocktake', in S. Gillam (ed) *What has New Labour done for primary care? A balance sheet*, London: King's Fund, pp 1-24.

Gladstone, D. (1995) *British welfare policy: Past, present and future*, London: UCL Press.

Glennerster, H. (1985) *Paying for welfare*, Oxford: Blackwell.

Godlove, C. and Mann, A. (1980) 'Thirty years of the welfare state: current issues in British social policy for the aged', *Aged Care and Services Review*, vol 2, no 1, pp 1-10.

Goldberg, T. and Connelly, N. (1982) *The effectiveness of social care for the elderly*, London: Heinemann.

Griffiths, R. (1983) *NHS management inquiry*, London: DHSS.

Griffiths Report (1988) *Community care: An agenda for action*, London: HMSO.

Hadley, R. and Clough, R. (1996) *Care into chaos: Frustration and challenge in community care*, London: Cassell.

Hadley, R. and Hatch, S. (1981) *Social welfare and the failure of the state: Centralised social services and participatory alternatives*, London: Allen and Unwin.

Harris, A. (1961) *Meals on Wheels for old people*, London: National Corporation for the Care of Older People.

Harris, A. (1968) *Social welfare for the elderly: Volume one, comparison of areas and summary*, London: HMSO.

Health Advisory Service (1983) *The rising tide: Developing services for mental illness in old age*, Sutton: Health Advisory Service.

Henwood, M. (1992) 'Twilight zone', *Health Services Journal*, 5 November, pp 28-30.

Heywood, F., Oldman, C. and Means, R. (2001) *Housing and home in later life*, Buckingham: Open University Press.

HM Government (1976) *An attack on inflation: A policy for survival: A guide to the government programme*, London: HMSO.

Hoggett, P. (1990) *Modernisation, political strategy and the welfare state: An organisational perspective*, DQM Paper No 2, Bristol: SAUS Publications.

House of Commons Social Services Committee (1985) *Community care with special reference to adult mentally ill and mentally handicapped people*, second report (Session 1984-85), House of Commons Paper 13-I, London: HMSO.

House of Commons Social Services Committee (1987) *Primary healthcare*, first report (Session 1986-87), House of Commons Paper 37-I, London: HMSO.

Hoyes, L. and Means, R. (1994) 'Open plan', *Health Services Journal*, 4 August, p 23.

Hoyes, L., Means, R. and Le Grand, J. (1992) *Made to measure? Performance measurement in community care*, Bristol: SAUS Publications.

Hoyes, L. et al (1993) *User empowerment and the reform of community care: A study of early implementation in four localities*, Bristol: SAUS Publications.

Hoyes, L., Lart, R., Means, R. and Taylor, M. (1994) *Community care in transition*, York and London: Joseph Rowntree Foundation and *Community Care*.

Hudson, B. (1990) 'Social policy and the New Right – the strange case of the community care white paper', *Local Government Studies*, vol 16, no 6, pp 15-34.

Hudson, B. (2000) 'Modernising social services – a blueprint for the new millennium', in B. Hudson (ed) *The changing role of social care*, London: Jessica Kingsley, pp 219-38.

Hunt, A. (1970) *The home help service in England and Wales*, London: HMSO.

Huws Jones, R. (1952) 'Old people's welfare – successes and failures', *Social Service Quarterly*, vol 26, no 1, pp 19-22.

Johnson, N. (1987) *The welfare state in transition: The theory and practice of welfare pluralism*, Brighton: Wheatsheaf.

Judge, K. and Sinclair, I. (1986) *Residential care for elderly people*, London: HMSO.

Kemp, M. (1973) 'An update on the workhouse', *Built Environment*, vol 2, no 9, p 496.

Kendall, J. (2000) 'The mainstreaming of the third sector into public policy in England in the 1990s: whys and wherefores', *Policy & Politics*, vol 28, no 4, pp 541-62.

Knapp, M., Hardy, B. and Forder, J. (2001) 'Commissioning for quality: ten years of social care markets in England', *Journal of Social Policy*, vol 30, no 2, pp 283-306.

Labour Party (2001) *Ambitions for Labour – Labour's manifesto 2001* (www.labour.org.uk).

Laing and Buisson (1992) *Care of elderly people market survey*, London: Laing and Buisson.

Laing and Buisson (1994) *Care of elderly people market survey*, London: Laing and Buisson.

Laing, W. and Saper, P. (1999) 'Promoting the development of a flourishing independent sector alongside good quality public services', in M. Henwood and G. Wistow (eds) *Evaluating the impact of caring for people*, Research Volume Three to the Royal Commission on Long-Term Care, Cm 4192, London: The Stationery Office, pp 87-102.

Langan, M. (1990) 'Community care in the 1990s: the community care White Paper, *Caring for people*', *Critical Social Policy*, Issue 29, pp 58-70.

Lart, R. and Means, R. (1993) 'User empowerment and buying community care: reflections on the emerging debate about charging policies', in R. Page and N. Deakin (eds) *The costs of welfare*, Aldershot: Avebury, pp 107-27.

Leach, S. and Wilson, D. (2000) *Local political leadership*, Bristol: The Policy Press.

Le Grand, J. and Bartlett, W. (eds) (1993) *Quasi-markets and social policy*, Basingstoke: Macmillan.

Lewis, J. (1993) 'Developing the mixed economy: emerging issues for voluntary organisations', *Journal of Social Policy*, vol 22, pt 2, pp 173-92.

Lewis, J. and Glennerster, H. (1996) *Implementing the new community care*, Buckingham: Open University Press.

Liberal Democrats (2001) *Freedom, justice, honesty: Liberal Democrat manifesto for disabled people* (www.libdems.org.uk).

Local Government Act (1999) London: The Stationery Office.

Lord Chancellor (1999) *Government policy on archives*, Cm 4516, London: The Stationery Office.

Lowe, R. (1999) *The welfare state in Britain since 1945* (2nd edn), Basingstoke: Macmillan.

Lund, B. (1999) '"Ask not what your community can do for you": Objectives, New Labour and welfare reform', *Critical Social Policy*, vol 19, no 4, pp 447-62.

Means, R. (1993) 'From Poor Law to the marketplace', in C. Grant (ed) *Built to last? Reflections on British housing policy*, London: Shelter Publications, pp 154-64.

Means, R. (1999) 'Housing and housing organisations: a review of their contribution to alternative models of care for elderly people', in A. Tinker et al, *Alternative models of care for elderly people*, Research Volume Two to the Royal Commission on Long-Term care, Cm 4192, London: The Stationery Office, Appendix 3, pp 299-324.

Means, R. (2001) 'Lessons from the history of long term care for older people', in J. Robinson (ed) *Towards a new social compact for care in old age*, London: King's Fund, pp 9-27.

Means, R. and Smith, R. (1985) *The development of welfare services for elderly people, 1939-71*, London: Croom Helm.

Means, R. and Smith, R. (1998a) *From Poor Law to community care: The development of welfare services for elderly people, 1939-71*, Bristol: The Policy Press.

Means, R. and Smith, R. (1998b) *Community care: Policy and practice* (2nd edn), Basingstoke: Macmillan.

Means, R., Morbey, H. and Smith, R. (2000) 'What is health care? What is social care? Shifting boundaries in four contrasting local authorities', in A. Dickenson, H. Bartlett and S. Wade (eds) *Old age in a new age*, Oxford: Oxford Brookes University, pp 181-5.

Mishra, R. (1984) *The welfare state in crisis: Social thought and social change*, Brighton: Wheatsheaf.

MoH (Ministry of Health) (1950) *Welfare of old people*, Circular 11/50, 23 January, London: MoH.

MoH (1957a) *Local authority services for the chronic sick and infirm*, Circular 14/57, 7 October, London: MoH.

MoH (1957b) HM (57) 86 *Geriatric services and the care of the chronic sick*, 7 October, London: MoH.

MoH (1959) *Report of the Ministry of Health for the year ended 31st December 1958*, Cmnd 806, London: HMSO.

MoH (1963) *Health and welfare: The development of community care*, Cmnd 1973, London: HMSO.

MoH (1965a) *The care of the elderly in hospitals and residential homes*, Circular 18/65, London: MoH, 20 September.

MoH (1965b) *Home Help Service*, Circular 25/65, London: MoH.

National Audit Office (1987) *Community care developments*, House of Commons Paper 108 (Session 1987-88), London: HMSO.

Parker, J. (1965) *Local health and welfare services*, London: Allen and Unwin.

Parker, R. (1988) 'An historical background', in I. Sinclair (ed) *Residential care: The research reviewed*, London: HMSO, pp 1-38.

Peace, S., Kellaher, L. and Willcocks, D. (1997) *Re-evaluating residential care*, Buckingham: Open University Press.

Pearson, G. (1983) *Hooligan: A history of respectable fears*, Basingstoke: Macmillan.

Phillips, D., Vincent, J. and Blacksell, S. (1988) *Home from home: Private residential care in Devon*, Sheffield: University of Sheffield and *Community Care*.

Phillipson, C. (1982) *Capitalism and the construction of old age*, Basingstoke: Macmillan.

Phillipson, C. (1998) *Reconstructing old age: New agendas in social theory and social policy*, London: Sage Publications.

Phillipson, C., Bernard, M., Phillips, J. and Ogg, J. (2001) *The family and community life of old people*, London: Routledge.

Plank, D. (1978) 'Old people's homes are not the last refuge', *Community Care*, 1 March, pp 16-18.

Player, S. and Pollock, A. (2001) 'Long-term care: from public responsibility to private good', *Critical Social Policy*, vol 21, no 2, pp 231-55.

Powell, M. (ed) (1999) *New Labour, new welfare state?*, Bristol: The Policy Press.

Powell, M. (2000) 'New Labour and the Third Way in the British Welfare State', *Critical Social Policy*, vol 20, no 1, pp 39-60.

Power, M. (ed) (1997) *The audit society: Rituals of verification*, London: Macmillan.

Pressman, J. and Wildavsky, A. (1973) *Implementation*, Berkeley: University of California Press.

Price Waterhouse/Department of Health (1991) *Implementing community care: Purchaser, commissioner and provider roles*, London: HMSO.

Prime Minister (1999) *Modernising government*, Cm 4310, London: The Stationery Office.

Propper, C., Bartlett, W. and Wilson, D. (1994) 'Introduction', in W. Bartlett, C. Propper, D. Wilson and J. Le Grand (eds) *Quasi-markets in the welfare state*, Bristol: SAUS Publications, pp 1-9.

Qureshi, H. (1999) 'Outcomes of social care for adults: attitudes towards collecting outcome information in practice', *Health and Social Care in the Community*, vol 7, no 4, pp 257-65.

Rao, N. (2000) *Reviving local democracy: New Labour, new politics?*, Bristol: The Policy Press.

Robinson, J. (ed) (2001) *Towards a new social compact for care in old age*, London: King's Fund.

Royal Commission on the National Health Service (1979) *The Merrison Report*, Cmnd 7615, London: HMSO.

Rudd, T. (1958) 'The home care of old people', *The Medical Officer*, 29 June, p 395.

Rummery, K. and Glendinning, C. (1999) 'Negotiating needs, access and gatekeeping: developments in health and community care in the UK', *Critical Social Policy*, vol 19, no 3, pp 353-70.

Scott, J. (1990) *A matter of record*, Cambridge: Polity Press.

Secretary of State for Health (2000a) *The NHS Plan: A plan for investment, a plan for reform*, Cm 4818-I, London: The Stationery Office.

Secretary of State for Health (2000b) *The NHS Plan: The government's response to the Royal Commission on Long-Term Care*, Cm 4818-II, London: The Stationery Office.

Seebohm Report (1968) *Report of the Committee on Local Authority and Allied Personal Social Services*, Cmnd 3703, London: HMSO.

Silverman, D. (1995) *Interpreting qualitative data: Methods for analysing talk, text and interaction*, London: Sage Publications.

Sinclair, I. and Williams, J. (1990) 'Domiciliary services', in I. Sinclair et al (eds) *The kaleidoscope of care: A review of research on welfare provision for elderly people*, London: HMSO, pp 159-78.

Slack, K. (1960) *Councils, committees and concern for the old*, Occasional Paper on Social Administration No 2, Welwyn: Codicote Press.

Social Services Inspectorate (1987) *From home help to home care: An analysis of policy, resourcing and service management*, London: DHSS.

Social Services Inspectorate (1988) *Managing policy change in the home help service*, London: DHSS.

Social Services Inspectorate (1989) *Towards a climate of confidence*, London: DoH.

Stake, R.E. (1995) *The art of case study research*, London: Sage Publications.

Sutherland Report (1999) *With respect to old age: The Royal Commission on Long-Term Care*, Cm 4192, London: The Stationery Office.

Taylor-Gooby, P. (2000) 'Blair's scars', *Critical Social Policy*, vol 20, no 3, pp 331-48.

Taylor, M. and Hoggett, P. (1994) 'Quasi-markets and the transformation of the independent sector', in W. Bartlett, C. Propper, D. Wilson and J. Le Grand (eds) *Quasi-markets and the welfare state*, Bristol: SAUS Publications, pp 184-206.

Thomas, D. and Means, R. (2000) 'Getting started: early research findings on a jointly managed community-based rehabilitation service', *Managing Community Care*, vol 8, issue 6, pp 41-4.

Tinker, A. (1997) *Older people in modern society* (4th edn), Harlow: Longman.

Townsend, P. (1962) *The last refuge*, London: Routledge and Kegan Paul.

Townsend, P. (1986) 'Ageism and social policy', in C. Phillipson and A. Walker (eds) *Ageing and social policy: A critical assessment*, Aldershot: Gower, pp 15-44.

Townsend, P. and Wedderburn, D. (1965) *The aged in the welfare state*, London: Bell.

Wagner Report (1988) *Residential care: A positive choice*, London: National Institute for Social Work.

Walker, A. (1981) 'Towards a political economy of old age', *Ageing and Society*, vol 1, no 1, pp 78-94.

Walker, A. (1989) 'Community care', in M. McCarthy (ed) *The new politics of welfare: An agenda for the 1990s*, Basingstoke: Macmillan, pp 203-24.

Warburton, R. and McCracken, J. (1999) 'An evidence-based perspective from the Department of Health on the impact of the 1993 reforms on the care of frail elderly people', in M. Henwood and G. Wistow (eds) *Evaluating the impact of caring for people*, Research Volume Three of the Royal Commission on Long-Term Care, Cm 4192, London: The Stationery Office, pp 25-36.

Warren, M. (1951) 'The elderly in the community', *Social Service Quarterly*, vol 24, no 3, pp 102-6, 120.

Wilcock, G. (1990) *Living with Alzheimer's disease and similar conditions*, London: Penguin.

Willcocks, D., Peace, S. and Kellaher, L. (1987) *Private lives in public places*, London: Tavistock.

Willcocks, D., Peace, S., Kellaher, L. and Ring, A. (1982) *The residential life of old people: A study in 100 local authority old people's homes*, Volume 1, Research Report No 12, London: Survey Research Unit, Polytechnic of North London.

Winchester, R. (2000) 'Everything up for grabs', *Community Care*, 9-15 November, p 12.

Wistow, G., Knapp, M., Hardy, B. and Allen, C. (1992) 'From providing to enabling: local authorities and the mixed economy of social care', *Public Administration*, vol 70, no 1, pp 25-46.

Wistow, G., Knapp, M., Hardy, B. and Allen, C. (1994) *Social care in a mixed economy*, Buckingham: Open University Press.

Wolfenden Committee (1978) *The future of voluntary organisations*, London: Croom Helm.

Working Group on Government Relations Secretariat/Local Government Association (2000) *Local compact guidelines: Getting local relationships right together*, London: National Council for Voluntary Organisations.

World Health Organisation (1992) *The ICD-10 classification of mental and behavioural disorders*, Geneva: World Health Organisation.

Index

NOTE: Page numbers followed by *fig* indicate information is contained in a figure, those followed by *tab* that information is in a table.

national standards for care 14, 18, 22, 24, 163-5
need assessment 150-7
New Labour *see* Labour government
New NHS, The (White Paper) 20
New Right theories 22-3
new service provision 114-16
NHS *see* National Health Service
nursing care/homes
  eligibility criteria 153, 154*fig*
  funding for 15, 145-50
  independent sector 59, 61-2, 145-50
  staff requirements in residential care homes 55-7, 84
  voluntary sector provision 60*tab*, 62
  see also independent sector residential care; residential care

P

Parker, J. 29, 166
partnership in health provision 21, 168
Patients first (consultation paper) 74
Pearson, G. 6
performance assessment 18, 24, 171-2
person-centred care 164*fig*
personal care
  costs of/funding for 15, 16*tab*, 164-5, 168, 169, 173-4
  definitions of 16*fig*
  in home care services 38-9, 43-4
  personal care plans 22, 148
Phillipson, C. 176
Plank, D. 38
planning
  corporate strategy 8, 10-11
  joint planning 75-6, 90-2, 107, 167
Player, S. 173
policy
  adverse effects of 3
  effect of resources on 11
  globalisation and 22, 23
  and health services 73-7
  residential care policy 64-8
  Third Way 13, 22-4
Pollack, A. 173
pooled budgets 20-1
Poor Law legacy 165-6

Powell, M. 23-4
Power, M. 24
primary care groups/trusts 20, 21-2
Priorities for health 75
prioritisation for funding 25, 39-45, 157
private sector *see* contract culture; independent sector; mixed economy approach; quasi-markets
Propper, C. 129-30
psychiatric care
  criticism of services 3, 91-2
  dementia cases 56-7, 90-2, 175
  hospital closures 80-1, 90
public assistance institutions 49-50, 52
public expenditure *see* funding/public expenditure
purchaser/provider split 77, 135-45, 155

Q

quality standards 137, 139, 142, 148-9, 163-5
quasi-markets 129-58
  competition between in-house and independent services 140-2
  Conservative introduction of 2, 5, 22-3, 24
  defining features 129-30
  independent sector 145-50, 174
  purchaser/provider split 77, 135-45, 155

R

race issues 175-6
reforms 2-6, 59, 129-58
  marketisation reforms 2, 5-6, 22-4, 25, 27-8
  see also mixed economy approach; modernisation agenda; quasi-markets
Registered Homes Act (1984) 61, 69
replacement programmes 111-12
research study outline 6-9
residential care
  capital investment in 50-4, 57-8, 166

staff
  for home care services 3, 44–5
  inadequate levels 3, 54–8, 84
  in post-war residential care homes
    50
standards for care 14, 18, 22, 24, 137,
    142, 148–9, 163–5
strokes 164*fig*
surveillance 24, 171, 172, 177
Sutherland Report 2, 14–16, 22,
    164–5, 168, 170

T

targeting of funds 25, 36–45
Taylor, M. 99
Taylor-Gooby, P. 23
teaching hospitals: detrimental effect
    82
Third Way policies 13, 22–4
time-limited grants 114–16, 117, 121
Towards a climate of confidence (quality
    recommendations) 63–4
Townsend, Peter
  on home help service 29–30, 33
  on residential care 50, 101, 166
transition funds 3

U

urban aid 115
user assessment 4, 150–7

V

verification ideology 24
visiting schemes 28–9
voluntary sector
  and contract culture 116–22
  funding for 29, 106–7, 107–8,
    114–17, 119–21
  historical involvement 29, 100–14
  and independent sector growth
    109–14
  joint finance develops role of 89,
    114–15
  in joint working process 94, 107–8
  meals on wheels service 102–5
  mixed economy approach 99–125

new service provision 114–16
nursing home provision 60*tab*, 62
range of services provided 102
residential care partnerships 111–12

W

Wagner Report 61
Walker, A. 5
Warburton, R. 170
Warren, M. 28
Wedderburn, D. 29–30
Willcocks, D. 61
Williams, J. 38–9, 45
Wistow, G. 132
Women's Royal Voluntary Service
    (WRVS) 100, 101
  meals on wheels provision 102–5
workhouse spectre 165–6
Working for patients (White Paper) 75
WRVS 100, 101, 102–5

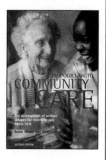
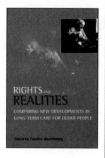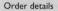